A Merciful End

A Merciful End

The Euthanasia Movement in Modern America

Ian Dowbiggin

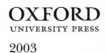

2003

OXFORD

UNIVERSITY PRESS

Oxford   New York
Auckland   Bangkok   Buenos Aires   Cape Town   Chennai
Dar es Salaam   Delhi   Hong Kong   Istanbul   Karachi   Kolkata
Kuala Lumpur   Madrid   Melbourne   Mexico City   Mumbai   Nairobi
São Paulo   Shangai   Taipei   Tokyo   Toronto

Copyright © 2003 by Oxford University Press, Inc.

Published by Oxford University Press, Inc.
198 Madison Avenue, New York, New York 10016

www.oup.com

Oxford is a registered trademark of Oxford University Press

Library of Congress Cataloging-in-Publication Data

Dowbiggin, Ian Robert, 1952–
A merciful end : the euthanasia movement in modern America/
Ian Dowbiggin.
p.   cm.
Includes bibliographical references and index.
ISBN 0-19-515443-6
1. Euthanasia—United States—History.   I. Title.
R726.D69   2002
179.7—dc21   2002022458

9 8 7 6 5 4 3 2 1

Printed in the United States of America
on acid-free paper

To Jamie,
joy and courage personified

Contents

Acknowledgments

In writing and researching this book I have amassed numerous debts. In particular, I wish to thank the Social Sciences and Humanities Research Council of Canada and the University of Prince Edward Island's Senate Committee on Research for their generous support. Stephen Berger, Donald Cregier, Donald Critchlow, Leslie Hall, Jeffrey House, Susan Martinuk, Randolph B. Schiffer, Richard Weikart, and Andrew Winston have helped me to clarify my thinking about the history of euthanasia. Dinah O'Berry of Lewis Advertising in Baltimore and David Klaassen at the Social Welfare History Archives at the University of Minnesota provided invaluable archival assistance. As always, Ginny Kopachevsky was indispensable when it came to electronic searches and interlibrary loans, as was the research performed by John Cusack and the day-to-day help offered by Anna Fisher and Deena Bugden of the University of Prince Edward Island's history department. I am also grateful to George Annas, Derek Humphry, Karen Orloff Kaplan, Mary Meyer, Donald McKinney, Timothy Quill, Ruth Roettinger, Ruth Proskauer Smith,

Margaret Somerville, and Marjorie Zucker for graciously consenting to be interviewed. Their willingness to discuss past and present betokens a refreshing openness, raising hopes that sooner rather than later a humane consensus on death and dying will take shape in America.

Introduction

On Sunday night, November 22, 1998, viewers of the CBS television program *60 Minutes* watched in horror as Dr. Jack Kevorkian killed fifty-two-year-old Thomas Youk. Youk, suffering from amyotrophic lateral sclerosis, or Lou Gehrig's disease, had asked Kevorkian to end his life, and Kevorkian complied by injecting him with poison to stop his heart.

Youk was not the first person Kevorkian had helped to die, but he was likely the last. In 1999, the seventy-year-old Kevorkian was convicted of second-degree murder and sentenced to jail for ten to twenty-five years.

What Kevorkian had done was deliberately and mercifully hasten another person's death, an act of active "euthanasia," taken from the Greek word for "easy death." Acquitted of the charge of assisting suicide by three juries in the 1990s, Kevorkian crossed the line in 1998 by not only administering the lethal injection but also videotaping Youk's death and defying prosecutors to charge him. Kevorkian's goal in life is to overturn America's laws prohibiting both active euthanasia and assisted suicide, in which someone purposely asks another (most often a physician) for help in dying. But by killing Youk, he very well might have done irreversible harm to his life's mission.

Kevorkian's conviction and the backlash it triggered are among the most recent in a long series of events stretching back to the nineteenth century that represent attempts by numerous men and women to change the nation's attitudes and laws about euthanasia. A handful, like Kevorkian, have resorted to sensationalist, open defiance of the law in the effort to gain acceptance of an individual's unlimited right to choose the time, manner, and place of his or her death. Others have tried a quieter approach, but they too have shared Kevorkian's conviction that they were engaged in a revolutionary struggle to free Americans from ethical codes of conduct that date back to classical antiquity. They have been united by their commitment to fighting for "the right not to suffer," whether because of unwanted pregnancy, deferred sexual gratification, or a lingering, painful death. Still others agree that Americans have every right to refuse unwanted medical treatment, but believe that such a right is entirely different from a right to have a physician either administer or prescribe lethal drugs to a terminally ill patient. Today, as in the past, Americans sharply disagree over what constitutes death with dignity, but very few think that the question of how we die should be a hidden secret.

This book, thanks to privileged access to confidential records of the euthanasia movement, is the first to chronicle how America reached this state of affairs. It tells the story of one of the most contentious yet neglected chapters in the history of American policy reform, a cautionary tale of a political, social, and cultural struggle that since its origins has been firmly embedded in the frequent and surprising twists and turns of broader history and now shows signs of raging well into the twenty-first century. We now know a great deal about Nazi medical killing between 1939 and 1945, a program that, in the name of euthanasia, ultimately cost the lives of some 100,000 handicapped adults and children. In recent years, there has also been extensive media coverage and analysis of the Netherlands' experiment since the 1970s with both physician-assisted suicide and active voluntary euthanasia, in which doctors or others directly end a consenting patient's suffering. But what little we know about euthanasia in modern America chiefly comes from those accounts that, in their partisan approach to sources, have left out much of its history and fostered myths that persist to this day. They have tended to depict euthanasia advocates as engaged in a triumphalist struggle between virtuous representatives of democratic rights and hidebound professional and religious institutions dedicated to defending their self-interests at the expense of individual freedom.

This book explodes both this myth and the other myth that the modern euthanasia movement began only in the 1960s and 1970s with the introduction of life-prolonging medical technology, the decline of the doctor-patient relationship, the rise of the "rights culture," medicine's inept handling of end-of-life care, and the AIDS epidemic. As important as these factors were, they simply helped to focus public attention on a century-old discourse, predating World War I, which affirms a theory of individualism stressing emancipation, independence, and autonomy. Euthanasia—or "the right to die," as the movement is more widely known today—certainly was popularized by shifts in medical technology or practice and truly became grassroots after the 1960s, but its ideological strands have long been entangled in the divisive cultural conflicts in America over what defines the boundaries between personal autonomy and public authority, between individual freedom and the notion of a common good.

Attention to the discourse of autonomy behind the euthanasia movement reveals, however, some disturbing paternalist tendencies. While most right-to-die advocates today stress that they seek only the freedom of competent, terminally ill individuals to choose medical assistance in dying, up to the end of the twentieth century various proponents have also expressed a worrying willingness to extend the legalization of euthanasia to cover persons with disabilities, handicapped newborns, and unconscious geriatric patients, or to justify the right to die for social and economic reasons. This combination of a fervent quest to maximize human freedom and the reformist urge to socialize individual identities in the service of utilitarian goals is as old as the Progressive era of the early twentieth century. The enduring nature of this current within America's euthanasia movement justifies the concerns of some, more recent, interested parties that legalizing physician-assisted suicide or active euthanasia will lead to a "reduction of respect for human life," ultimately affecting the disabled and other vulnerable persons in society. The right to die can all too easily become "a duty to die."[1]

At the same time, however, there is little historical evidence that the right-to-die movement in America, if unchecked, will lead inevitably to genocide, as some alarmists believe. This line of argument is based on comparisons between the history of the euthanasia movement in the United States and what transpired in Nazi Germany. Comparisons between German and American euthanasia are not illegitimate; indeed, given the stark contrast between the enormous scholarly literature on Nazi euthanasia and the meager literature on Anglo-American euthanasia, they are long overdue. In fact, American euthanasia proponents from time to time have uttered statements that share a troubling similarity with those of German physicians before and after Hitler. However, such comparisons run the risk of confusing many important distinctions that emphasize the uniqueness of Nazi medicalized murder and the exceptionalism of American political culture, with its repeated invocations of personal liberty and freedom of choice, to say nothing of its robust religiosity. "Playing the Nazi card" also potentially poisons the chances of a reasoned debate over a health care question that at the turn of the twenty-first century is far more complex than was the case in the war-torn Third Reich.[2] Not every slope is slippery, and not all medical abuse is tantamount to Nazism.

The history of American euthanasia thus confirms what scholars such as Donald T. Critchlow have argued, that the complexity of the process leading to reform and policy change does not lend itself to a neat division between "good guys" and "bad guys."[3] This is particularly true in the early twenty-first century, as Americans try to ignore the rhetoric and grapple with the hard questions posed by the myriad ethical, social, cultural, and economic conditions surrounding death and dying.[4] As the physician Sherwin Nuland contends, nothing needs to be demythologized more than the process of dying and the concept of death with dignity, if Americans are to avoid the self-deceptions and disillusionment that inevitably result from not knowing the truth.[5] This book provides a historical perspective on society's long struggle to deal with the grim reality of human disintegration that we call death.

Chapter 1 charts the history of euthanasia as both a concept and a practice from classical antiquity to the Progressive era. Before World War I, the overwhelming consensus among Americans was that physicians were justified in trying to provide their dying patients with a "easy death" by making them as comfortable and pain free as possible, but there was almost no public support for legalizing active mercy killing. Only when the popularity of social Darwinism, scientific naturalism, eugenics, positivism, and the ideology of Progressivism mounted at the beginning of the twentieth century, undermining faith in traditional religious beliefs, did a debate begin over whether or not the state should permit painless killing of incurable patients.

Euthanasia first became a topic of national controversy in 1915 when a Chicago surgeon refused to operate on a deformed baby and thus allowed it to die. The extensive press coverage of this case revealed that there was a growing minority of educated Americans, some of them Progressives convinced of the need to apply scientific theory to social problems and conventional values, who were inclined to let defective infants die as a humane way of curtailing human breeding, thus reducing the number of unfit individuals in society.[6]

However, euthanasia remained a marginal social issue until the Depression. In 1938, the Euthanasia Society of America (ESA) was founded, the first national organization in favor of legalizing mercy killing and the focus of chapter 2. The ESA tried mightily to nudge popular opinion increasingly toward an acceptance of active euthanasia. Against a backdrop of growing debate over euthanasia in the 1930s, and the founding of a similar organization in England, the founders of the ESA brought to the new organization valuable experience acquired through participation in the eugenics, women's suffrage, and birth control campaigns. Many ESA members were convinced that with the vote for women won, the decriminalization of birth control imminent, and the enactment of eugenic sterilization laws in the 1920s, the next victory would be the legalization of active euthanasia. They tended to believe that death would be the last taboo to fall in the struggle to free Americans from what birth control activist Margaret Sanger, herself an ESA member, called "biological slavery."

Chapter 3 follows the ESA's history from the Depression to the 1960s, a time when the ESA *was* the American euthanasia movement. These were years when ESA officials became mired in a culture war with the Roman Catholic Church over euthanasia as well as birth control, a conflict over what they viewed as the unconstitutional power of the established churches to dictate their values to all American citizens. The ESA leadership spent these years on the defensive, trying to free the group from any association with the Nazi euthanasia programs, but its failure to erase the Nazi taint crippled its attempts to convince state legislators to enact laws giving consenting adults the right to a medically administered death. The ESA's battle with the Catholic Church, waged within a cultural climate dominated by anticommunism and heightened religiosity, ended in defeat, and euthanasia advocates would spend much of the 1960s devising new strategies for winning over popular opinion.

Changes in strategy paid off by the late 1960s. As chapter 4 shows, during that decade the ESA reinvented itself as a organization dedicated to passive rather than active euthanasia, the right to refuse unwanted treatment rather than the right to a medically administered, speedy death. Public interest in death, spurred by the writings of Elisabeth Kübler-Ross and others, became a virtual "craze" by the 1970s, as Americans celebrated the end of "the conspiracy of silence" surrounding death. Thanks to the help of the advice columnist "Dear Abby" and the introduction and distribution of "living wills" (advance directives written by individuals specifying under what conditions treatment would be withheld), the ESA capitalized on the constitutional recognition of a right to privacy and the sixties' emphasis on individual choice. Euthanasia ceased being defined as active mercy killing, with its disturbing overtones of coercion and social usefulness, and increasingly became viewed as personal freedom *from* unwanted interference in one's own life. This redefinition of euthanasia benefited enormously from the rise of the women's movement in the 1960s, with its celebration of "our bodies, ourselves." As society's traditional caregivers, women all too often have watched their spouses, parents, children, and friends die, and thus the notion of preventing unnecessary suffering has had special meaning for them. The women's movement, blossoming in the sixties and seventies, provided a nurturing environment for the revived euthanasia movement.

Yet even in a cultural climate stressing personal choice, right-to-die advocates never totally rejected utilitarian justifications for euthanasia. In the 1960s and 1970s, the ESA attracted wealthy backers of population control such as the tycoon Hugh Moore and philanthropist John D. Rockefeller 3rd, and the idea spread that euthanasia was the responsible thing to do in an overpopulated world of diminishing resources.

Success crowned the ESA's efforts to redefine euthanasia as a right to refuse unwanted medical treatment in the 1970s and 1980s, when state after state legalized living wills and money poured into the group's coffers from a sympathetic public. The massive press coverage surrounding the tragic story of Karen Ann Quinlan, who lapsed into an irreversible coma in 1974, put a human face on the right to die in ways that all the ESA's official literature could never do. But just as the movement seemed poised to make the big breakthrough to the legalization of active euthanasia, its unity began to crumble, as chapter 5 shows. The ESA itself underwent various name changes and split into two factions during the 1970s, a sign of the creative ferment, quiet reflection, and acute disagreements among euthanasia advocates. Tensions abruptly developed between radicals interested only in winning the legal right to active euthanasia and physician-assisted suicide, and a growing number of moderates who believed that the issues surrounding death and dying were far more complex than earlier imagined and warranted further study and public discussion. These fault lines hardened with the founding of the World Federation of Right-to-Die Societies and Derek Humphry's grassroots Hemlock Society in 1980. By then, the center of gravity for the entire euthanasia movement was shifting from the East Coast to the West Coast, from the fashionable and affluent Manhattan locations where the ESA's board used to meet to the drafty and damp church basements where the rank-and-file ("little old Ohio ladies in running shoes," as one activist described them) of the new, populist right-to-die organizations congregated to hammer out policy.

The momentum of the 1980s led to fierce legal and legislative battles over the right to die in the 1990s. The poignant fate of Nancy Cruzan highlighted the plight of families faced with difficult end-of-life decisions. Ballot initiatives in three states in the early 1990s came close to winning the right to die with medical assistance, and victory was finally achieved in 1997 when Oregon became the first American state to permit physician-assisted suicide. Overseas, as the decade drew to a close, Belgium and the Netherlands enacted analogous legislation allowing doctors to help patients die, after the Dutch had tolerated the practice since the 1980s. Thoughtful individuals such as the physician Timothy Quill supported assisted suicide as a regrettable yet indispensable "last resort" in palliative care. By the end of the 1990s, international and national trends seemed to indicate that euthanasia enjoyed public backing as never before.

In the 1990s, however, as interest in palliative care, pain management, and hospice treatment spread, other organizations were formed, dedicated to care for people at the end of life, but highly skeptical of the need for legalizing active euthanasia or physician-assisted suicide. Similar views were expressed by the 1994 New York State Task Force on Life and the Law, which supported the long-standing argument that a legal right to die would diminish respect for life. An energized and politically savvy right-to-life movement, spearheaded by the Roman Catholic Church, also mobilized stiff opposition to the right to die by linking euthanasia and abortion. Revulsion over Jack Kevorkian's well-publicized assisted suicides tarnished the euthanasia movement's credentials. In 1997, the Supreme Court ruled that there is no constitutional right to die, and Congress's 1999 bill outlawing the use of narcotics to cause death jeopardized the Oregon law. In 1998 and 2000, the voters of Michigan and Maine, respectively, voted against legalizing physician-assisted suicide, demoralizing defeats for right-to-die proponents.

Thus, while trends in Europe in favor of legalizing euthanasia appear strong at the beginning of the twenty-first century, and opinion polls in the U.S. record wide public support for a right to die, many Americans continue to believe that legalizing either active euthanasia or assisted suicide would be bad public policy. Heartbreaking personal stories about people dying difficult deaths in cold and impersonal hospitals rarely fail to elicit widespread public sympathy, but when Americans are asked to endorse changing current laws to permit euthanasia, a majority still balks. There appears to be a diffuse willingness to tolerate the practice of assisted suicide and active euthanasia in individual cases, and few Americans oppose the legal right of competent adult persons to refuse unwanted treatment, but the consensus seems to be that laws barring euthanasia should remain in place because the potential dangers of a dramatic change in public policy regarding euthanasia would outweigh any benefits from its legalization. The upshot of this state of affairs for the American euthanasia movement by the early twenty-first century is that, though its history since the nineteenth century suggests it has come a long way, a major victory continues to elude its supporters.

The prospects for such a victory also look dim. As even stalwarts such as Derek Humphry reluctantly agree, the battle over euthanasia in coming years will be long and drawn out, with no conclusive outcome in sight. Right-to-die proponents show few signs of climbing down from the barricades, but neither do their opponents, who are no longer confined to the ranks of the Christian Right or right-to-life groups. The future of the euthanasia movement will ultimately depend on how the debate over self and society unfolds in the present century, how the tension between the search for a boundless individualism and the quest for a meaningful community is resolved. Above all, the prospects of victory for the right-to-die movement will be dictated by the broad course of American history itself and the nation's shifting political culture. Until a clear winner emerges in these cultural "wars," the right to die will be what it was for much of the twentieth century: a fiercely contested reform that sparks strong passions as do few other issues.

A Merciful End

1

Origins

How do we save civilization? physician William Duncan McKim asked rhetorically in 1900. A "gentle, painless death" for America's drunkards, criminals, and people with disabilities was his answer. The only thing that stood in the way, McKim explained, was the "unreasonable dogma that *all* human life is intrinsically sacred." The march of science, he concluded, dictated that Americans give up this long-standing religious belief.[1]

McKim's secular and scientific rationales for euthanasia in the early twentieth century signaled a revolutionary challenge to literally hundreds of years of Judeo-Christian teaching about the dignity of human life. For centuries, euthanasia had normally been understood to mean the process whereby the relief of pain for the dying was the best way to ensure an "easy death." However, that changed in the late nineteenth century when euthanasia acquired its modern connotation. For the first time in history, people began defining it as actual mercy killing.[2]

Thanks to radically new currents of thought during the second half of the nineteenth century, a handful of Americans such as Mc-

Kim began to entertain the idea that humanely hastening the death of hopelessly ill persons, or "active" euthanasia, was acceptable policy and not a criminal act. Trends such as eugenics, positivism, social Darwinism, and scientific naturalism had the effect of convincing a small yet articulate group in the early twentieth century that traditional ethics no longer applied to decisions about death and dying.[3] These Americans, often identified with other reform causes such as birth control and women's suffrage, disputed the doctrine that life was primarily a sacred gift from God, and that there was something inherently redeeming or noble about suffering. This evolution in thought, when combined with the Progressive movement between the 1890s and the 1930s, led to the first calls in American history for a "natural right to a natural death." The awkward Progressive mix of humanitarianism, idealism, statism, faith in naturalist science, respect for the "gospel of efficiency," and belief in social control nurtured the first stirrings of interest in euthanasia, but it also bequeathed its uneasy compound of liberal and illiberal motives to later generations of right-to-die supporters.[4] The Progressive era would set the stage for the emergence in the 1930s of an organized euthanasia movement, and its effects on the right-to-die debate would still be felt a half-century later.

I.

As Alexis de Tocqueville observed in the 1830s, there was no nation more Christian than the United States on the face of the earth, and at the beginning of the twentieth century this was as true as ever.[5] Many Americans took a casual attitude toward the finer points of Christian theology, but the vast majority of American Protestants and Roman Catholics agreed that the Bible was binding on elementary issues of doctrine and practice.[6] American Jews thought similarly.[7] The overwhelming belief was that the commandment "thou shalt not kill" proscribed mercy killing.

However, in ancient Greece and Rome, before the coming of Christianity, attitudes toward infanticide, active euthanasia, and suicide had tended to be tolerant. Many ancient Greeks and Romans had no cogently defined belief in the inherent value of individual human life, and pagan physicians likely performed frequent abortions as well as both voluntary and involuntary mercy killings. Although the Hippocratic Oath prohibited doctors from giving "a deadly drug to anybody, not even if asked for," or from suggesting such a course of action, few ancient Greek or Roman physicians followed the oath faithfully. Throughout classical antiquity, there was widespread support for voluntary death as opposed to prolonged agony, and physicians complied by often giving their patients the poisons they requested.[8]

These values and practices clashed sharply with Judaic and Christian beliefs about suicide and the inherent value of life.[9] Like Judaism, Christianity teaches that God endowed human life with intrinsic value. From the first century A.D. to the twentieth century, virtually all Christians condemned suicide as a means of escaping the suffering that afflicts human beings. This accounted for the uniformity of opinion throughout Christendom about the virtues of extending human life and enduring suffering when death approached as an essential part of God's providential plan for each and every individual. Throughout the New Testament and the writings of the Church Fathers, the lesson is clear: Failure to resign oneself to the will of God in the final act of life amounts to a breach of trust in God and a rejection of God's gift of life.[10]

There was a remarkable continuity in Church medical ethics regarding suicide and euthanasia between the dawn of Christianity and the late Middle Ages. Medieval references to voluntary death were rare, suggesting that the actual practice of euthanasia had tapered off dramatically since the fall of Rome. Laws in some parts of Europe dictated that a suicide's corpse be dragged through the streets or nailed to a barrel and left to drift downriver. The medieval ethos was distinctly uncongenial to any kind of self-murder.[11]

Even the coming of the Renaissance and Reformation did not fatally weaken Christian condemnation of suicide and euthanasia.[12] However, during the eighteenth-century Enlightenment, a tiny handful of European intellectuals, including Voltaire, Montesquieu, and David Hume, expressed tolerant opinions about suicide and euthanasia.[13] The word "suicide" replaced the term "self-murder," a change evident by the early eighteenth century.[14] The questioning of the prohibition against suicide was part of the Enlightenment celebration of science as an alternative to clericalism and orthodox Christian doctrine. Similarly secular doubts about the taboo against euthanasia would be expressed in the twentieth century.

However, Enlightenment toleration of suicide proved to be temporary. Under the leadership of evangelicals such as John Wesley, a vigorous religious counterattack gained momentum as the late eighteenth century drew to a close. The various waves of religious revivalism, starting with the Great Awakening of the mid-1700s, prevented secularists and agnostics on either side of the Atlantic Ocean from generating popular support for taking one's life. These events dovetailed with the Second Great Awakening of intense evangelical fervor in the first years of the nineteenth century and strengthened the condemnation of suicide and euthanasia that stretched back to the earliest days of colonial America.

The rejection of suicide and euthanasia remained firm, even after many of the new states decriminalized suicide in the wake of the Revolutionary War.[15] The majority of Americans rejected suicide's common-law punishment, namely, forfeiture of the suicide's estate and an ignominious burial, both of which were widely seen as a cruelty to the suicide's family. But no matter how sympathetic they were toward the suicide's family, most Americans stopped far short of condoning self-murder. As late as the antebellum period there existed in the United States a firm consensus, informed by centuries of Judeo-Christian teaching, against suicide and mercy killing. Nineteenth-century Americans viewed both practices—but especially mercy killing—as rebellion against God's will and outrages against the sanctity of human life.[16]

II.

This moral consensus held firm as nineteenth-century physicians, buoyed by breakthroughs in diagnostic precision and inspired by a new philosophy regarding treatment, increasingly became the dominant figures in the death chamber, asserting their responsibility to provide physical and moral comfort to the dying. Despite the harrowing scenes physicians sometimes witnessed of patients dying in grave pain, and the fact that sometimes doctors performed active euthanasia to ease the suffering of patients and their families, very few Americans before the twentieth century felt that there was a need to legalize euthanasia.[17]

To doctors for most of the nineteenth century, the lesson seemed to be that palliating pain at the time of death was more humane than using every possible means to prolong life. Increasing numbers of physicians questioned the effectiveness of their traditional therapies, such as bleeding and purging, and accepted the idea that doing less rather than more for their patients freed up nature's healing powers to effect a cure. This skeptical approach to therapeutics actually empowered physicians, enabling them to assert their indispensable role in managing the care of the dying patient, instead of fighting tooth and nail to postpone death. In an era when most Americans died at home rather than in a hospital and were often surrounded by friends and relatives, the doctor emerged as an important figure in the family circle, there to soothe and comfort the patient with words and (if necessary) doses of alcohol, opium, or morphine. The doctor's job was to make the terminal stage easier for everyone, patient and loved ones alike. It was not only to produce a peaceful, easy, and painless death but also to participate in a religious ceremony that represented death as a long-awaited end to the "pilgrimage through the wilderness of the world," a departure from the sadness and pain of temporal existence, with the bliss and glory of heaven awaiting. Religion and medicine blended at bedside, highlighting the physician's success in dispensing effective terminal care.[18]

However, revolutionary developments in French scientific medicine in the first half of the nineteenth century challenged this image of the doctor tending to the dying. French clinicians recorded patients' symptoms and then matched them with autopsical observations, a mode of inquiry that, combined with heavy reliance on statistical studies, enabled doctors to classify specific diseases. With diagnosis and prognosis more exact, physicians were able for the first time in history to know with fair probability whether a patient was unlikely to recover. Under the influence of French medical teaching, American physicians began believing they could predict the outcome of a disease and determine whether or not it was incurable. This knowledge meant they could now propose active euthanasia with a clearer conscience.[19]

Similarly, by the Civil War, the introduction of analgesics, anesthesia, and the hypodermic administration of morphine made it possible for physicians not only to relieve severe suffering due to disease but also to ease dying patients painlessly across the River Styx. Under these circumstances, some physicians committed active euthanasia, using chloroform or narcotics "to plunge the patient into a profound sleep, whence he may or may not come forth."[20] As a University of Buffalo surgeon stated in 1913,

I know that others have assumed the responsibility, which I myself have taken in more than one case, of producing euthanasia, when, in the terminal stage of life, a patient was suffering the tortures "of the damned," and has pleaded for a method of escape, the pleadings being seconded by the family. Under these circumstances I think that to administer a lethal dose of morphine or of chloroform is to "do as one would be done by."[21]

However, then, as later, doctors—while willing to admit they faced occasions in which mercy killing was indicated—were generally reluctant to discuss whether they actually performed active euthanasia. Nor, in the end analysis, was there a glaring need for such a practice. In an age before life-prolonging, artificial feeding machines, those patients in permanently unconscious states, unable to either eat or drink, would eventually pass away. Even when patients lingered in pain from illnesses such as cancer, they often contracted pneumonia ("the old man's friend") and died sooner rather than later. The suffering of dying patients was something all doctors witnessed from time to time, but death appeared to be near enough in most cases to obviate the need for active euthanasia.[22]

If anything, organized medicine's opposition to active euthanasia became stronger near the end of the nineteenth century as physicians grew more therapeutically optimistic. Hospitals ceased being charitable and religious institutions for poor and dying patients and became medical institutions dedicated to curing disease and the scientific study of illness. Surgery, thanks to the introduction of anesthesia and aseptic techniques, was transformed into a respectable medical specialty that could be performed on a variety of conditions, such as appendicitis, gall bladder disease, stomach ulcers, and—most important—cancer.[23] Patients generally shared this confidence in medicine's power to cure. These rising expectations of doctors' authority and therapeutic capabilities by the early twentieth century would plateau in the 1960s and 1970s, but until then patients' faith in American physicians remained strong.[24]

Thus, public confidence in medicine's ability to cure disease tended to undercut any support for euthanasia among physicians. Citing the danger of "bring[ing] the profession into discredit," physicians' organizations in America and England vigorously opposed the right of individuals to seek medical help in ending their lives.[25] Significantly, on the few occasions when euthanasia was advocated, it was nonphysicians who usually did so.[26] As Abraham Jacobi, a pioneer in the study of childhood diseases, asked rhetorically in 1912: "Would a doctor who would consent to satisfying the suggestions of the people who clamor for 'Euthanasia' ever again deserve the confidence of the public?"[27] American doctors insisted that their task was to cure disease, save lives, and ease suffering, not "don the robes of an executioner."[28] Highly dependent on public confidence, doctors overwhelmingly shared their society's moral values. If most physicians would not support birth control before the 1960s because it clashed with Americans' sense of right and wrong, they were even less likely to endorse euthanasia.[29] Before doctors and their patients could accept euthanasia, a profound change in the country's moral sentiments was necessary.

III.

The two great revolutions before the 1960s that affected Americans' attitudes and expectations regarding euthanasia were the late-nineteenth-century growth of scientific knowledge and the coming of Progressivism. Each trend in its own way helped to undermine orthodox religious faith, question the authority of tradition, and engender a taste for daring social experimentation in the name of justice, efficiency, public health, and human emancipation. Progressivism, a response to the fundamental social and economic changes during the first decades of the twentieth century—including urbanization, industrialization, mass immigration, labor unrest, racial tensions, mobilization for world war, and the exploitation of the country's natural resources—solidified faith in science as both a method of inquiry and a type of knowledge that might help social scientists and policymakers manage such changes efficiently while easing the hardship of countless Americans. Armed with this reverence for science and technocratic expertise, Progressives became not only receptive to previously heretical ideas such as eugenics and euthanasia but also increasingly disposed to interpret euthanasia as a form of social control. Progressives often viewed euthanasia as a public health measure designed to minimize the costs of supporting disadvantaged groups, improve the welfare of future generations, and reconstitute the basis for an enduring social order. Progressives were inspired by humane motives, but their strong belief in elite, scientific leadership also meant that their paternalistic methods would often compromise the democratic goals they claimed they sought. Later champions of the right to die would inherit from the Progressives this same tension between methods and motivations, "conscience and convenience," the search for personal autonomy and the quest for community through expert-led social engineering. Many would insist they supported euthanasia as a means to achieve individual freedom, but their interpretations of a right to die had little to do with the pioneer individualism of nineteenth-century Americans. Instead, they took a page out of the neoprogressive writings of philosopher John Dewey and cast the freedom to choose death as both a fundamental right and an exercise in socialization that, in an age of dizzying change that threatened to subvert personal autonomy, restored the fragile relationship between self and society. Euthanasia, in this view, was less a regrettable last resort than a desirable use of one's democratic citizenship.[30]

Before the coming of Progressivism, the foundations of the American euthanasia movement were laid by the remarkable trends in the natural and social sciences in the late nineteenth century. Biblical criticism, originating in Germany and subjecting the Scriptures to rigorous historical scrutiny, encouraged the belief that the Bible was more inspirational literature than revealed truth. The discovery of the second law of thermodynamics, in stating that energy was not created and existing energy was gradually dissipating, cast doubts on the notion of a kindly and benevolent Providence. In the face of these developments, growing numbers of educated Americans started to believe that conventional moralism was useless in the face of the modern realities facing the country by the turn of the twentieth century.[31]

The most pivotal turning point in the early history of the euthanasia movement was the coming of Darwinism to America. By calling into question "the most foundational beliefs of Americans, almost all of which derive from the Judeo-Christian tradition," Darwinism contributed significantly to the "major crisis of faith" that climaxed in the 1920s with the Scopes "Monkey" trial in Dayton, Tennessee.[32] As John Dewey announced in 1909, Darwin "introduced a mode of thinking that in the end was bound to transform the logic of knowledge, and hence the treatment of morals, politics, and religion."[33] Numerous American intellectuals agreed with Dewey, saying that reading Darwin had changed their lives by shaking their faith in Christianity, its claims to transcendental truth, and its code of ethics and morality. Many Christian thinkers complained that, in light of

Darwin and the theories of his follower Herbert Spencer, "the old sanctions of morality are all undermined."[34] It is likely that some personal Anglo-American testimonials to the impact of Darwinism on religious faith were retrospective rationalizations of intellectual changes that had been years in the making and pre-dated the publication of *The Origin of Species* in 1859.[35] However, to many Americans, the teaching of Darwinism meant science ought to replace religion as the arbiter of social policy and ethical conduct. What often replaced faith in the old gods was a belief that truth was relative, itself a product of historical and natural process.

In the *Origin of Species* and *Descent of Man* (1871) Darwin explained his theory of evolution according to natural selection, effectively demolishing the reigning school of "natural theology" in Anglo-American biology. Natural theology taught that the complexity and intricacy of the living world proved there had to be a God who, in separate acts of creation, had fitted each species with the traits that enabled it to adapt to its particular environment.[36] Darwin instead argued that species were not independently created but were descended from a common ancestor. Species were modified throughout natural history because the fierce struggle for limited food supply weeded out the unfit individuals of a species and privileged the fit, which by surviving tended to pass on their favorable traits to offspring. This process of "natural selection" accounted for the modification of species and was even sufficient to bring about new species. Thus, there was no "design" or divine purpose in nature, nor were species fixed and discrete entities. The immense variety in the organic world was due to natural laws that the "Creator" had "impressed" on matter on the day when evolution began. Becoming an evolutionist, as historian Ronald Numbers has contended, did not necessarily mean rejecting all acts of special creation, and it did not mean accepting everything Darwin wrote; but it undermined the overall theory of special creation.[37]

Long before writing the *Origin of Species*, Darwin had believed that the human race was part of evolution, but in the *Origin* he was extremely careful to say nothing about the matter.[38] In his 1871 *Descent of Man*, Darwin threw caution to the wind, affirming boldly that "man is the co-descendant with other mammals of a common progenitor."[39] With that statement, Darwin declared that the human mind—and by implication the soul—rather than being prior to things, was emergent in nature. Mind was naturalized, and for philosophers such as Dewey, this was the most revolutionary message of the theory of evolution. After Darwin, it was perfectly logical to conclude that the moral instinct in human beings was a product of natural selection and there were no immutable laws governing ethical behavior. The roots of human moral consciousness lay in man's nonhuman ancestry. This, and much else, made the *Descent of Man* a greater threat to Judeo-Christian morality than the *Origin*.[40]

What replaced the standard Christian code of morality was unclear, and on this score Darwin himself was little help.[41] Later thinkers filled in this gap in Darwinian theory, however, unambiguously defending a form of ethical relativism that said what individuals decided to do could be judged only in terms of the situational circumstances surrounding a particular act.[42] Not surprisingly, some post-Darwinian intellectuals exploited such reasoning to justify suicide and euthanasia. Whether people decided to kill themselves depended on the situation in which they found themselves. Absolute standards were irrelevant to the uniqueness of individual existence.

Robert G. Ingersoll, the lawyer and outspoken agnostic, was the first to defend a right to euthanasia by exploiting these implications of Darwinism. Ingersoll maintained that morality "is the best thing to do under the circumstances," and the best thing to do under the circumstances was "that which will increase the sum of human happiness—or lessen it the least."[43] Born in 1833, in Dresden, New York, Ingersoll at an early age rebelled against the orthodox Christianity of his Congregationalist minister father. He went on to champion such iconoclastic causes as feminism, birth control, and racial tolerance. The nineteenth century was "Darwin's century," Ingersoll proclaimed, and the churches, in trying to fight Darwinism, were simply obstructing the march of truth. "You cannot harmonize evolution and the atonement," Ingersoll declared. "The survival of the fittest does away with original sin."[44]

Ingersoll's reverence for Darwinist science and his interest in revising traditional morality also explains his respect for positivism, the teaching of the French philosopher Auguste Comte (1798–1857). Positivism was the belief that the human race had evolved through two stages of development by the nineteenth century. The first stage was the theological one, when people tended to attribute all natural phenomena to the acts of gods. The second was the metaphysical stage, when people ceased invoking gods and instead believed in abstract theories divorced from observation. Comte announced that the nineteenth century would inaugurate a new stage, in which individuals would subscribe to the positive philosophy, the notion that all the sciences (including the social sciences) should be based on rigorous observation and the scientific calculation of the mathematical laws that governed the world. Equipped with such knowledge, Comte predicted, society would be able to harness these laws for the prosperity and progress of the human race. For such insights, Ingersoll stated, Comte "will be lovingly remembered as a benefactor of the human race."[45]

Positivism's veneration of science, progress, and social reorganization, as well as its assault on superstition and bigotry, appealed to Ingersoll as it did to numerous American liberals in the late nineteenth and early twentieth centuries. Comte's positivism served as a kind of bridge between the naturalism of the late nineteenth century and the liberalism of the Progressive era, a discourse that played a large role in the origins of the euthanasia movement. Twentieth-century liberals' statist and corporatist bent, as well as their confidence in reform, government interventionism, and technocratic elites, can be traced back to the Comtean tradition of the previous century.[46]

Armed with his belief in Darwinism and positivism, Ingersoll repudiated the Christian concept of God, the Bible as the inspired word of God, Christ as a divine being, and the dogma of hell and damnation. He saw his mission in life to be the liberation of the human mind from the alleged ignorance, prejudice, and cruelties of religion. Science not only represented truth; it also offered the tools and techniques for human beings to fulfill their destinies on earth. As individuals, people could construct their own ethical codes and patterns of conduct based on observation, experience, and reason, regarding life from a purely "natural point of view."[47]

Given Ingersoll's eagerness to dispute most of Christian orthodoxy, it was little wonder that he took an unconventional approach to the question of suicide. Although he never advocated suicide as a way of avoiding difficulties in life, he saw it as a rational choice in hopeless cases such as terminal cancer. In 1894 he created a great stir when he defended a right to suicide. A man "being slowly devoured by cancer," suffering acutely and in agony, "is of no use to himself" nor his wife, children, friends, and society. He is actually a "burden to himself and to others, useless in every way," and thus enjoys the "right to end his pain and pass through happy sleep to dreamless rest." If there was a benevolent God, Ingersoll added, he could take no pleasure in the suffering of such people.[48]

It is worth examining Ingersoll's thought closely because, in its essentials, it differs little from justifications of euthanasia many years later when changes in medical technology had supposedly made active euthanasia an urgent necessity. Ingersoll's utilitarian theory that whatever maximizes human happiness is best is remarkably similar to twentieth-century Humanism, the ideology of the American Humanist Association (founded in 1942). Humanists, who believe that giving individuals the widest freedom of choice over personal life and death matters is the best way to reduce the sum of human misery, and that science ought to be privileged over religious knowledge, have been at the forefront of the movement to legalize euthanasia in modern America. Like later Humanist rationales for euthanasia, however, Ingersoll's definition of life maneuvered uneasily between vindicating individual choice in defiance of established moral guidelines and passing sweeping judgments about what constituted "useful" life. He never adequately distinguished a right to die from the notion that in certain situations it might be right for some unfortunate individuals to die. Even an adamant libertarian such as Ingersoll was guilty of saying who did and did not deserve to live.

Ingersoll's views resembled those of Felix Adler, in 1891 the first prominent American to openly endorse suicide for the chronically ill. Adler, like Ingersoll, welcomed the appeal to recast conventional religious ethics and morality. He did so by fashioning a new and nondogmatic approach to religion that, in emphasizing ethics over doctrine, echoed Ingersoll's adamantly secular approach to moral conduct. The founder of the Ethical Culture movement in 1876, Adler was born in Germany in 1851 and moved to the United States in 1857 with his family. He returned to Germany to complete his rabbinical training, but during his stay in Germany he became disenchanted with Judaism. Upon his return to America in 1873, he called for the universalization of the Jewish religion, stressing morality over piety or adherence to a particular set of beliefs. "Diversity in the creed, unanimity in the deed," he stated in 1876. "This is that practical religion from which none dissents." He called this new version of Judaism "Ethical Culture" and proposed it as a common ground on which people from different faiths and walks of life could unite.

Unlike Ingersoll, Adler did not reject religion. He simply tried to revolutionize American religion through Ethical Culture, the teaching that religion is nothing more than ethics. But, whatever their original differences, during the course of the twentieth century Ethical Culture and Humanism became so alike that they were almost indistinguishable, especially on the issue of euthanasia.[49]

Adler never succeeded in revolutionizing American religion, but before he died in 1933, he had founded numerous kindergartens, schools, settlement houses, and study groups that spread the teaching of Ethical Culture and drew followers from reform Judaism and liberal Christianity. His defense of suicide to escape the suffering of death also left a mark on history because it forged the striking and close kinship between Ethical Culture and the euthanasia movement in the twentieth century. In 1891 Adler argued that chronic invalids should hold out for as long as possible, but when their pain and unhappiness became overwhelming they deserved the right to die peacefully. Adler urged that such a process, if legalized, be rigorously safeguarded and voluntary; if it were, the attending physician should be permitted to administer "a cup of relief."[50]

Adler's interest in euthanasia was only tangential to his chief reform concerns, such as child welfare, public nursing, slum improvements, and vocational training. Nonetheless, as exemplified by Ethical Culture Society members who supported euthanasia in later years, there was a vital philosophic link between Ethical Culture and mercy killing. Adler stressed that human beings were made up of two natures, the spiritual and the physical. The physical part of human nature is the means, and the spiritual part is the end. "The physical life is *not* to be preserved if by preserving it we deny or defeat" the spiritual part, Adler warned. To him, there was a grave danger in investing the physical side of a person with "the sacred character that belongs to the spiritual."[51]

In constructing this argument, Adler anticipated the thinking of later defenders of euthanasia who contended that when the ravages of disease and disability compromised the integrity of an individual's personality and quality of life, suicide was not just permissible—it was rational and humane. To Adler and his followers, who were sympathetic to the notion of suicide when death beckoned, there was no absolute value assigned to life. If life was not sacred, Adler, like Ingersoll, believed that some lives were less worth living than others. Both insisted that individuals should enjoy the freedom to do with their lives what they wished, even if it meant killing themselves. However, by rejecting the old taboos against suicide and euthanasia, they left the door open for many of their followers in the twentieth century to stretch their definitions of mercy killing to include individuals other than competent, consenting adults.

IV.

Ethical Culture's chief impact on the euthanasia movement would be delayed until later in the twentieth century. In the meantime, late-nineteenth-century Americans such as Ingersoll pounced on Darwinism because its purely naturalistic interpretation of human experience seemed to call into question absolute moral standards that, they believed, stood in the way of progress and the alleviation of hardship. They also liked Darwinism because it seemed so readily applicable to the study of society. Followers of Darwin, such as Herbert Spencer and William Graham Sumner, eloquently made the case for what came to be called "social Darwinism." In the words of the Darwinist president of the American Association for the Advancement of Science in 1887: "Questions of labor, temperance, prison reform, distribution of charities, religious agitations are questions immediately concerning the mammal man and are now to be seriously studied from the solid standpoint of observation and experiment and not from the emotional and often incongruous attitude of the church." Empirical and experimental science, in the form of evolutionary biology, should therefore guide social policy.[52]

Darwin himself was a social Darwinist of sorts. In his *Descent of Man*, he argued that civilization in the form of asylums, hospitals, public charity, and therapeutic medicine obstructed the power of natural selection, enabling the "weak members" of society to survive and reproduce their own kind. Worse, "the reckless, degraded, and often vicious members of society, tend to increase at a quicker rate than the provident and generally virtuous members." To Darwin, this meant the "degeneration" of the human race was a distinct possibility. If late-nineteenth-century society wanted to make progress an "invariable rule," he warned, it had to prevent "the reckless, degraded, and vicious" from reproducing.[53]

Darwin personally shrank from endorsing the draconian policy implications of these gloomy thoughts, hoping vaguely that the unfit would voluntarily refrain from marriage and the fit would have big-

ger families. However, many of his defenders were not so ambivalent. They preached the need for social measures that would prevent
the sick, maimed, and mentally handicapped from breeding, lest
their fertility lead to race degeneration. Thus, eugenics was born.
Between the Gilded Age and the 1960s, when the word "eugenics"
went out of fashion, the histories of the eugenics and euthanasia
movements would be closely intertwined.[54]

The term eugenics was coined in 1883 by Darwin's cousin, the
Englishman Francis Galton, from the Greek for "wellborn." Galton
defined eugenics as "the science of improving stock," including the
use of "agencies of social control" to "improve . . . the racial qualities
of future generations."[55] With its emphasis on social planning, preventive medicine, and the study of heredity, the theory of eugenics
swept across much of the globe over the next half-century, affecting
science, medicine, and public health policy. Governments from Sweden to Latin America introduced legislation based on eugenic principles, including laws restricting marriage, curbing immigration, and
permitting coercive sterilization of the handicapped. Eugenics authorized the reduction of social problems to utilitarianism and evolutionary biology while dispensing with approaches based on traditional value systems, largely what many advocates of euthanasia
were inclined to favor. Little wonder that, over the first half of the
twentieth century, the fledgling euthanasia movement would recruit
many of its members from the ranks of eugenic organizations.[56]

By the 1920s, the United States had become perhaps the world's
most eugenic nation. Most of America's geneticists, biologists, physicians, and social scientists had embraced eugenics, a trend that
culminated in the founding of the American Eugenics Society in
1923.[57] Eugenics pervaded college, university, and high school curricula. The Carnegie and Rockefeller Foundations funded eugenic
research. In 1921 and 1924, Congress, influenced by eugenic arguments in favor of reduced immigration, passed legislation establishing nationality quotas for newcomers to the United States.[58] By the
1930s, forty-one states had laws prohibiting marriage of the mentally
ill and the mentally retarded, and thirty states had passed eugenic
sterilization laws.[59] Eugenics would fall out of favor after World War
II, largely due to Nazi Germany's own 1933 eugenic sterilization law,
but until then eugenics enjoyed the support of a broad segment of
educated opinion in the United States.

Eugenics in America was not limited to debates among biologists about social policy. Its cultural meaning extended far beyond the science of genetics to encompass public health concerns such as diet, exercise, parenting, pediatrics, and personal hygiene. Although self-styled "serious" eugenicists disliked its popularization, evident in "better baby contests" and "eugenic" movies and stage dramas about the dangers of sexually transmitted diseases, the fact that eugenics had spread to the mainstream of American life testified to its powerful resonance as a weapon in the campaign to improve the nation's public health. As a method of preventing illness, eugenics spoke to the sensibilities of many early-twentieth-century Americans committed to making the country a healthier place to live, marry, and raise families. It would also speak to those who, in the coming years, viewed euthanasia as both an individual right and a socially beneficial practice.[60]

The growing cultural popularity and scientific acceptance of eugenics, coupled with social Darwinist views, led some Americans to question various aspects of traditional religious teaching. Following Galton, many American eugenicists evinced a spirit of antagonism toward religious orthodoxy. To some, eugenics was a surrogate religious doctrine.[61] Eugenicists such as Albert Wiggam, later a member of the Euthanasia Society of America, contended in 1923 that eugenics was a critical part of a revolutionary scientific worldview that "demands . . . a new set of values by which and for which to live," a "new code of conduct."[62] The eugenicist sociologist Frank Hankins, also a future member of the ESA, similarly proclaimed that the coming of eugenic birth control signaled an age of science when people were trying to "release the human spirit from the bondage of ignorance and superstition, taboos and fears."[63]

More cautious eugenicists, such as the psychologist and Clark University president G. Stanley Hall, disliked going as far as Wiggam did in testing all conventional guidelines according to the standards of science. They sought instead to reconcile Christianity with the march of eugenic theory. However, their ultimate loyalties lay more with evolutionary naturalism than Christianity. For figures such as Hall, if eugenics and evolution conflicted with the religion of their ancestors, then religion had to give way.[64]

The combined impact of eugenics and social Darwinism stimulated interest in euthanasia in early-twentieth-century America. By making the distinction between biological fitness and unfitness credible, these theories prompted Americans to reconsider conventional sentiments toward the handicapped, diseased, and underprivileged. This process had begun as early as 1877, when the American merchant Richard L. Dugdale highlighted the baneful effects on family history when individuals gave themselves up to crime, alcoholism, depravity, and pauperism.[65] Similar conclusions cropped up among medical professionals engaged in the study and care of the mentally retarded. By the early 1880s a consensus had emerged that state schools for the retarded were primarily designed to keep them from reproducing. Physicians, relying on the now-discredited theory that "like begets like," stressed both heredity and the high fertility of feebleminded girls. Incarceration and custodialism replaced rehabilitation. Segregation of the mentally retarded was viewed as desirable chiefly because it served eugenic purposes, which in turn saved governments money.[66]

The specter of spiraling costs to hospitalize the feebleminded, the insane, and other handicapped groups encouraged some Americans to broach the previously unmentionable idea of mercy killing the feebleminded and insane. This option was sometimes referred to as the "lethal chamber," drawing on the analogy to the room or receptacle in which animals were put to death painlessly through the use of poisonous gas.[67] Anticipating the intimate links between eugenics and euthanasia that would materialize in later years, a handful of Americans and Europeans began to ponder openly who should not be born and who was better off dead. In 1888, a delegate to the National Conference on Charities and Corrections revealed that, when he asked an unnamed Harvard-trained Boston physician, "what shall be done with this problem of the feebleminded? . . . He had a solution ready. It is a solution you have heard before. . . . He said, 'I would stamp out and kill the whole brood.' " Thoughts such as these almost always originated with social scientists or physicians who did not work with the mentally retarded.[68] However, when these minority views did surface, they were often couched in the language of Darwinism, eugenics, and the social benefits of taking such action. As one child welfare author argued in 1912, "cripples, high-grade cretins, idiots, and children with gross deformities" ought to be "quickly and painlessly destroyed." In particular, infanticide, with or without parental consent, was indicated when it was obvious which children would never "become useful members of society," or were "directly harmful to the species."[69]

The years on either side of 1900 witnessed a flurry of interest in these types of eugenic euthanasia. In addition to W. Duncan McKim, various Americans recommended selective infanticide, discouraged surgeons from operating on physically defective infants, called for mercy killing epileptics, alcoholics, and burglars, and urged gassing "the driveling imbecile."[70] Arguments such as these prompted a state representative in Ohio to introduce a bill, the first of its kind in American history. The Ohio bill permitted the killing with narcotics or anesthetic drugs of mature, consenting adults, "suffering enormous pains, that could not be relieved otherwise." The state legislature voted to send the bill to committee, where it died. However, the publicity surrounding the bill also sparked calls for eugenic-inspired laws that covered the mercy killing of the mentally handicapped and deformed children.[71]

The advent of Progressivism by this juncture in the country's history lent an air of urgency and respectability to such calls. Progressivism was the anxious response of the nation's educated elite to the enormous social, economic, and political changes that had overtaken the American people in the early twentieth century. In the quarter-century before 1914, eighteen million newcomers entered the United States, fomenting ethnic tensions and creating unprecedented problems for the country's social services. Industrial unrest accompanied this trend, as deplorable working conditions sparked strikes and violent responses from management. Huge discrepancies of wealth, most visible in the salaries of magnates Andrew Carnegie and J. P. Morgan, appalled people of conscience. Discontent with the economy motivated 900,000 Americans to vote for socialist Eugene Debs in 1912. Dissatisfaction with the lack of women's rights drove thousands of suffragettes to campaign for the vote. Racial tensions mounted as discrimination against blacks became institutionalized throughout the South. The release of D.W. Griffith's *The Birth of a Nation* in 1915 with its flagrant stereotyping of American blacks coincided with the resurrection of the Ku Klux Klan.[72]

Amid this unsettling strife and acute hardship, Progressives worked diligently to improve conditions. Grounds for optimism could be found in medical researchers who were discovering the microbes responsible for infectious diseases. Vaccines for diphtheria and syphilis were developed. The first modern hospitals devoted to research and treatment were being built.[73] Surgery was becoming safer and more successful. Public health measures improved sanitation and hygiene in America's burgeoning urban areas. Food purity

laws and labor legislation protecting the health and welfare of workers were passed, while governments invested heavily in schooling,
public nursing, and the prevention of juvenile crime.[74]

At the same time, thoughtful and concerned Americans, watching
massive urbanization, industrialization, immigration, and technological innovation steadily break down the old society of small towns
and isolated, rural communities, resolved to replace it with a new
and more viable social order.[75] Convinced that they lived in "a time
of unprecedented peril and opportunity" and waving "the flag of
generosity and conscience," Progressives united behind "a common
vision of a society happier because social engineers had brought an
end to wastefulness and irrationality in its various activities."[76] Progressive physicians, businessmen, scientists, engineers, academics,
and social workers looked toward the state and government bureauc-
racies to take active roles in reducing the incidence of poverty, disease, prostitution, alcoholism, or crime.[77] This Progressive reaction
to the nation's social problems embraced eugenics as a mainstream
reform, especially state sterilization laws.[78] Interest in euthanasia was
swept up in this general enthusiasm for eugenic and other public
health measures aimed at addressing the needs of the community
and those of its sick, disabled, and dying citizens. Eugenics mirrored
the Progressive ambivalence between benevolence and social control, as did early support for euthanasia.

William J. Robinson, a socialist, urologist, sex radical, and Progressive era muckraker, epitomized the links between eugenics and
euthanasia in 1913. Robinson was one of the earliest examples of
that common twentieth-century phenomenon, the left-leaning proponent of euthanasia who also campaigned for eugenics and birth
control, while urging society to adopt new value systems regarding
sex, birth, and death. Robinson utterly rejected the notion of individual liberty in cases of hereditary defectives or deformed infants.
"Such individuals have no rights," he contended in 1922. "They have
no right in the first instance to be born, but having been born, they
have no right to propagate their kind." He had no doubts that in
denying them these rights he was doing what was best for them as
individuals.[79]

It was not so much that Robinson thought that euthanasia was a
particularly effective eugenic tool; in fact he endorsed infanticide
mainly because doing so publicized society's failure to legalize contraception. Instead, his backing of euthanasia was tied to eugenics

because of his willingness to rank human beings differently in terms of their quality of life and imagined usefulness to the community. Not all human life was equal to him. Anticipating the arguments of later pro-euthanasia ethicists, Robinson argued that "[l]ife is sacred when it is pleasant, when it is wanted, when it is bearable. But a life of pain, agony, and anguish is not sacred, no more than a life of crime, shame, disgrace, and humiliation." Euthanasia was less important to him as a strictly eugenic measure than as a social policy that seemed to sanction revolutionary new moral attitudes toward formerly taboo topics.

Robinson concluded that exercising the euthanasia option was a sign of evolution in action. Humans who found themselves in acute pain during the last stages of life were employing the reason with which natural selection had endowed them when they chose assisted suicide "consciously and deliberately." Euthanasia, then, was more than a choice; under the proper circumstances, it separated humans from the rest of the animal kingdom and testified to their evolutionary superiority. Robinson, like many of his successors in the euthanasia movement, had difficulty separating the freedom to choose death from the evolutionary duty to die.[80]

Another notable Progressive-era American whose approval of euthanasia was mixed with an admiration of Darwinism, eugenics, and scientific naturalism was the novelist Jack London, author of the best-sellers *Call of the Wild* (1903) and *The Sea-Wolf* (1904). In 1913, three years before his death, London declared that a man's only true freedom was "anticipating the day of his death." London was a socialist, like Robinson and labor leader and founder of the American Socialist Party Eugene Debs, who also expressed his support for safeguarded euthanasia.[81] London's thinking, laced with heavy doses of Anglo-Saxon racialism, had been revolutionized by his reading of Darwin and Herbert Spencer, but he reserved a special fondness for the writings of Ernst Haeckel (1834–1919), the German biologist, eugenicist, social Darwinist, and euthanasia advocate.[82] Following Haeckel, London was a self-confessed materialist and atheist, rejecting the more moderate agnosticism of other Darwinians. "I have always inclined toward Haeckel's position," he wrote in 1914.

In fact, "incline" is too weak a word. I am a hopeless naturalist. I see the soul as nothing else than the sum of the activities of the organism plus personal habits, memories, experiences of the organism. I believe that when I am dead, I am dead. I believe that with my death I am just as much obliterated as the last mosquito you or I smashed.[83]

For London, euthanasia was a logical conclusion for someone like himself, persuaded that evolution and scientific naturalism were true. In a universe governed by the law of "nature red in tooth and claw," civilization's moral constraints often worked against evolution and had to be jettisoned when they clashed with the Nietzschean supermen who, in London's view, were society's natural leaders and thus above the law. Not surprisingly, London considered himself one of these supermen.[84]

London's esteem for Haeckel suggests that he had few qualms about the German philosopher's endorsement of euthanasia for Darwinist and eugenic purposes. Although he couched his support for euthanasia in terms of a personal "right to cease to live," an individual's freedom to choose how and when one was to die, London's heavy intellectual debt to Haeckel predisposed him to favor the killing of "helpless incurables" for the good of society or the species.[85]

Similar Progressive, eugenic, and naturalist themes also converged in the career of E. A. Ross. Ross, who would later serve on the ESA's advisory council, was one of the Progressive era's most esteemed social scientists, a professor of sociology at Stanford University and the University of Wisconsin. Ross's greatest contribution to the discipline of sociology was his book *Social Control*, published in 1901.[86]

Rejecting his religious upbringing after reading Darwin and Herbert Spencer, Ross in the late 1880s hailed Auguste Comte's positivist "religion of humanity" for the way it authorized a revamped system of values. For social scientists such as Ross, Comte's positivism was a beacon flashing amid the gloomy crisis he and others imagined wracked turn-of-the-century America. Positivism, with its high estimation of science and its prescriptions for social planning, held out the hope that the labor conflict, racial tensions, and disorienting pace of change in Progressive-era America could be reconciled with the obvious material improvements in medicine and science.[87]

Amid these raucous and unsettling times, Comte's philosophy appealed to Ross because of its apparent ability to harmonize progress and order. It enabled Ross and others, undergoing a personal crisis of faith in their parents' religion, to construct a "new liberalism," in Dorothy Ross's words, emphasizing "social control" exercised by technocratic experts as the means for ensuring further progress, without the disorder that seemed to accompany industrial expansion. Adherence to positivism provided Ross and like-minded Comteans with a "secular surrogate for traditional faith and piety."[88] Ross never recorded why he supported euthanasia, but his attraction to Darwinism, Progressivism, positivism, and eugenics suggests strongly that he, like William Robinson, believed conventional morality needed to be reassessed in light of the amazing new discoveries of science and the disquieting historical path America appeared to be choosing. Whatever religious creeds or ethical taboos could not withstand the glaring scrutiny of positivist science had to be rejected—and that included the sanctity of life.

These views spanning the years of the Progressive era underscore the point that American support for euthanasia was inspired more by shifting ideas, attitudes, and social forces than changes in medical practice or technology. Before World War I, no great breakthroughs had been made by medicine that prolonged dying unnecessarily, and thus could be used to justify the need for a right to die, as would be the case after the 1960s.[89] Whatever methods had been devised to make the hastening of patients toward death speedier and less painful were far outweighed by the progress in curing illness through bacteriology, surgery, or just better hospital care. Ingersoll, Adler, London, Ross, and Robinson themselves never cited the effects of medical innovations on death and dying as reasons for defending a right to die. Interest in euthanasia during the Progressive era relied instead on an elementary philosophic position that emphasized the need to construct new value systems, due to the revolutionary implications for traditional moral conduct of Darwinism, eugenics, positivism, scientific naturalism, and Progressive social improvisation. Robert Ingersoll was one of the very first to defend this viewpoint, but just as certainly he was not the last.

Still, in the years leading up to World War I, few predicted that Ingersoll's and Adler's ideas would have much impact. They were isolated figures within a cultural climate that emphatically rejected suicide, a condemnation that extended to the different types of euthanasia.[90] Medical opposition to euthanasia was firmly resolute. Euthanasia appeared to be the exclusive interest of a tiny minority, utterly out of step with the rest of American society. As a British observer wrote in 1906, America was the "land of hysterical legislation," where every now and again [the legalization of euthanasia] is put forward by literary *dilettanti* who discuss it as an academic subtlety or by neurotic "intellectuals" whose high-strung temperament cannot bear the thought of pain. The medical profession has always sternly set its face against a measure that would inevitably pave the way to the grossest abuse and would degrade them to the position of executioners.[91]

However, events would shortly confirm that euthanasia's appeal as a Progressive cause was considerably more complex and far-ranging than foreigners imagined.

V.

In the early hours of 12 November 1915, at Chicago's German-American Hospital, Anna Bollinger gave birth to her fourth child, a seven-pound baby boy. Her pregnancy had been uneventful and her labor fairly brief. However, the attending physician quickly noticed that the baby was blue and badly deformed. After conferring with the father, the doctor awakened Harry J. Haiselden, the hospital's forty-five-year-old chief of staff. Haiselden diagnosed a litany of physical defects, the most serious being no anal aperture. He predicted that, without surgery to construct an artificial anus, the child would die shortly from auto-intoxication.

In a decision whose shockwaves would ripple from coast to coast, and mark a milestone in the history of euthanasia in America, Haiselden advised against surgery. The Bollingers tearfully agreed and, on 16 November, Haiselden called a news conference to announce that, rather than operate, he would "merely stand by passively" and "let nature complete its bungled job." The child died on 17 November, amid growing controversy.

By declining to operate, Haiselden, born in 1870 in Plano, Illinois, almost singlehandedly managed to accomplish what other defenders of euthanasia before him had not. He not only got more Americans than ever before talking about euthanasia but also won endorsements from numerous prominent figures. The publicity surrounding his professional conduct, briefly eclipsing news from World War I, inspired other Americans to speak out in favor of letting deformed infants die for the good of society. A Progressive himself, Haiselden demonstrated how support for euthanasia was nurtured by a cultural climate punctuated by science, naturalism, and humanitarian reform.

Haiselden's decision not to operate was not an isolated incident in his career. He never revealed exactly how many infants he had allowed to die before the Bollinger incident, although he admitted it was many. In the three years after 1915, he was complicit in the deaths of at least five more abnormal babies. Rather than retire into the shadows of private life, Haiselden sought the limelight. He openly declared (incorrectly, as later researchers proved) that defective people were more fertile than normal individuals, although it is hard to see how anyone as crippled as the Bollinger boy could have grown up to spawn offspring.[92] Eugenic appeals to restrict immigration to specific national groups and prohibit marriages between people with hereditary illnesses won his hearty approval. He also admitted to performing eugenic sterilizations on several boys and girls upon the request of their parents.[93]

But Haiselden was an excellent example of how genuinely humane motives could co-exist with explicitly social and illiberal aims in the minds of euthanasia proponents. By 1915, he had lost faith in the custodial segregation of the mentally retarded, claiming that anything was better than letting children such as the Bollinger boy grow up and be housed in deplorable conditions. This helps to explain why he, a lifelong bachelor, adopted two daughters. He saw himself rescuing them from the wards of the nation's charity institutions. His affection for babies, deformed or healthy, was sincere and something that garnered praise from the press. In the eyes of many, he may have been a moral monster, but the real Haiselden was far more complex.[94]

As historian Martin Pernick has argued, distinctions among humane, Progressive, and eugenic motives made much less sense to Americans in Haiselden's day than they did to later generations. In advocating euthanasia for defective babies, Haiselden saw no incompatibility between serving the human race and doing what he thought was right for the child's sake. When it came to eugenics, there was no fundamental difference between the interests of society and the child's right not to suffer.[95] As he told the press in 1915, either the Bollinger baby dies after six days, or the nation is saddled with the costs of taking care of it and its offspring, none of whom would enjoy life anyway.[96]

Haiselden treated the eugenic issue surrounding the Bollinger story as a personal crusade. He was similar to Jack Kevorkian and the anarchists of his own day in that all of them practiced "a propaganda of the deed."[97] Haiselden exploited the available media of Progressive-era America, welcoming reporters onto hospital maternity wards to interview mothers and photograph their disabled babies. He wrote articles for Hearst newspapers, delivered public lectures, and posed for movie newsreels—all in the cause of highlighting the virtues of withholding treatment from defective infants. He also collaborated with a muckraking Hearst journalist, writing and starring in a feature motion picture titled *The Black Stork*. A eugenic dramatization of the Bollinger case, *The Black Stork* opened in 1916 to mixed reviews but continued being shown around the country until at least 1928.

Haiselden's eugenic characterization of euthanasia sensationalized what had happened to the Bollinger baby. "Eugenics? Of course it's eugenics," Haiselden explained to a reporter who had asked him about his decision not to operate. Underlining the close affinity between eugenics and euthanasia in early-twentieth-century America, some eugenicists by World War I had decided that mercy killing the disabled was an overdue reform.[98] Before 1915 the consensus among the leaders of the eugenics movement, including Karl Pearson, Harry H. Laughlin, Paul Popenoe, and Roswell Hill Johnson, was that euthanasia of the unfit was unwise and useless. But only a few months after the Bollinger baby died, the eugenicist Madison Grant argued that "the elimination of defective infants" was the welcome first step in "the obliteration of the unfit."[99] Other eugenicists, such as Yale economist Irving Fisher and biologist Charles Davenport, who dismissed euthanasia as a eugenic measure before 1915, defended Haiselden in the wake of the Bollinger incident. By taking a radical position on an already contentious issue, Haiselden made it easier for comparative moderates such as Fisher and Davenport to break their silence. Thanks to Haiselden's extremism, their views, although still controversial, suddenly looked much less heretical. It would not be the last time in the history of America's euthanasia movement that its grandstanding, Kevorkian-like militants would make formerly radical opinions appear mainstream.[100]

Haiselden's support also came from Americans who adhered closely to the Progressive faith that science, medicine, technology, and expert opinion could improve the lives of Americans dramatically. Haiselden enjoyed the backing of settlement worker Lillian

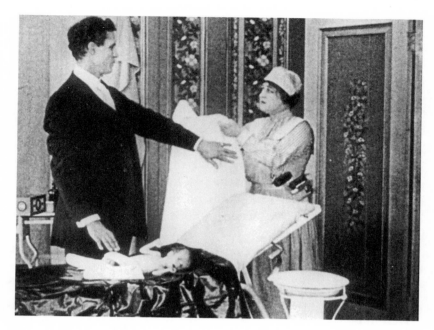

Harry Haiselden in a scene from the pro-euthanasia movie *The Black Stork*, reproduced in Martin S. Pernick's *The Black Stork: Eugenics and the Death of "Defective" Babies in American Medicine and Motion Pictures Since 1915* (Oxford and New York: Oxford University Press, 1996). *John E. Allen.*

Wald, Food and Drug Administration founder Harvey Wiley, birth control advocates such as William J. Robinson and his son Frederic, sex reformers such as Mary Ware Dennett and family law pioneer Judge Ben Lindsey, socialists such as Victor Robinson (William's son and Frederic's brother) and Anita Block. Helen Keller, the renowned advocate for the blind and deaf, approvingly equated Haiselden's campaign for euthanasia with Margaret Sanger's birth control crusade. Clarence Darrow, the civil rights lawyer, whose notoriety would peak in the 1920s during the Leopold and Loeb and Scopes "Monkey" trials, applauded Haiselden's actions when he declared: "Chloroform unfit children. Show them the same mercy that is shown beasts that are no longer fit to live."[101] Haiselden himself not only fit the description of a Progressive reformer, he also professed emancipated opinions for his time. He supported birth control and demonstrated a remarkable race-blindness when he hired an African-American surgeon for the German-American Hospital. Haiselden liked to compare his own campaign for euthanasia with the abolitionists' struggle against slavery.[102]

Haiselden had his critics, of course. Noted Progressives such as Julia Lathrop and Jane Addams denounced him for his refusal to operate on the Bollinger baby, proving that, while Progressivism disposed someone to sympathize with euthanasia, not all Progressives were euthanasiasts—nor were all euthanasiasts Progressives. The fact that many Progressives were inspired by the "social gospel" made them less liable to jettison Judeo-Christian morality in cases such as the Bollinger controversy. The majority of American physicians took the position that the doctor's first responsibility was to save lives, and that physicians who tried to determine who was and was not unfit to live were claiming a right that did not belong to them. Under the law, Haiselden was guilty for failing to perform his duty as a doctor to save or preserve life, so the nation's attorneys generally sided with the law and condemned Haiselden for violating the Bollinger baby's constitutional right to life.

The debate over Haiselden in the lay press was as diverse as the country itself. One St. Louis newspaper editorialized that Haiselden himself was a "moral defective," but other papers praised him for his humane intentions and for trying to save society money by letting disabled infants die. The liberal *New Republic* defended Haiselden by accusing his opponents of hypocrisy when they invoked the sacredness of life:

> This happens to be a nation which cannot boast that it cares supremely about babies, for hundreds of thousands of them die every year of preventable causes. They die of tenements which could be ventilated, of milk that could be kept clean, of neglect that could be remedied. They die because their fathers are underpaid, because their mothers are overworked; they are run over on city streets because there are insufficient playgrounds; they are infected by dirt diseases; they are starved. Given a chance in life most of them would become happy and even useful. They are refused that chance because public opinion is too indolent, because many landlords and businessmen are too greedy, because politicians are cowardly and ignorant. Every year hordes of human beings are condemned to death because

it costs too much to save them. But the refusal to keep alive a deformed idiot has become a moral issue throughout the nation.[103]

The *New Republic*'s editors agreed with Helen Keller that at issue was the definition of life, and that a right to life ought to be honored only when a potential for happiness, intelligence, and social usefulness existed. Tolerating "anomalies" such as the Bollinger baby, Keller wrote in the *New Republic*, "tends to lessen the sacredness in which normal life is held."[104]

Most Roman Catholics disagreed vehemently with Keller's line of reasoning and Haiselden's decision not to operate. It was precisely when babies such as the Bollinger infant were not tolerated that the belief in the sanctity of life declined, they argued. Besides betraying his trust to preserve life, Haiselden had played God by denying the Bollinger baby life and had thereby made further abuse possible. "[W]ho in the future will be safe" and "where will the line be drawn between the 'fit' and the 'unfit,' between the so-called 'defective' and 'non-defective'?" asked the newspaper for the Archdiocese of New Orleans.[105] In a version of what Catholics called the "wedge argument," another Catholic asked, "How long will it be until the weak-minded, the deformed, the infirm, and the aged will be disposed of according to the same theory?"[106] Haiselden's eugenic characterization drew the criticism that he had reduced human life to the ethics of "the Stud Farm and Cattle Pen."[107] Haiselden's defender Anita Block retorted by accusing the Church of being "eager to have millions of idiots and imbeciles born, so long as it can only get them baptized." Block and her Catholic foes agreed on precious little, but they were united in rehearsing the bitter conflict between euthanasiasts and the Church that would mark the remainder of the twentieth century.[108]

However, Catholic condemnation of euthanasia was not as absolute as it may have looked. The Church extolled suffering for its redemptive value, but it recognized that not all individuals could or ought to withstand suffering equally. It was not sinful for a physician who, seeking to minimize the pain of a patient in agony through narcotics, ended up killing the patient with an overdose. To Catholic ethicists, the intention of the doctor was crucial: If the aim was purely to relieve pain, then the act was not murder. This principle of the "double-effect," reaffirmed in a speech by Pope Pius XII in

1957, would remain central to Catholic teaching throughout the twentieth century and draw the criticism of euthanasia advocates who saw it as mere casuistry.[109]

Not all Catholics denounced Haiselden. Baltimore's James Cardinal Gibbons maintained that Haiselden was permitted to withhold surgery in the Bollinger case because such an operation would have been "extraordinary" treatment and hence optional. Other Catholics disagreed, insisting that the creation of an artificial anus was an "ordinary" procedure, but whatever debate there may have been among Catholics about what constituted "ordinary" or "extraordinary" treatment, all rejected Haiselden's eugenic justification.[110]

Support for Haiselden, then, did not necessarily mean approval of eugenics or mercy killing. Nor did opposition to Haiselden necessarily mean rejection of all types of euthanasia. Hugh Cabot, professor at Harvard Medical School, advocate for socialized medicine, and later vice president of the ESA, attacked Haiselden, but privately he favored euthanasia for his own family members and for incurably ill people who were not even suffering from severe pain.[111] Cabot was just one example of how some of the interested parties in the Bollinger drama interpreted Haiselden's conduct in ways that blur customary dividing lines. Many physicians in the twentieth century would demonstrate a similar inconsistency by either secretly helping patients to die or discontinuing treatment while publicly opposing euthanasia. The bare act of allowing a disabled newborn to die ordinarily would not have sparked so much controversy. It was Haiselden's public insistence that he refused to operate for chiefly eugenic reasons that transformed his behavior into a *cause célèbre*. His eagerness to mix eugenics and euthanasia set a pattern of provocativeness that would be followed by other euthanasiasts in later years, making the chances of staking out common ground all the more remote.

Thus, the fault lines that would emerge with greater clarity during the fierce disputes over euthanasia in the 1940s and 1950s were already evident during the Bollinger baby scandal. On the one side, Catholics and orthodox Protestants were gradually forging a position that condemned either elective or coercive mercy killing or the withholding of lifesaving medical treatment without the consent of the patient. They were united in their insistence that life was a sacred gift from God, and anyone who deliberately took human life was committing a grave sin against divine-inspired natural law. On the other side, a loose coalition was just beginning to form, made up of Americans who expressed varying degrees of sympathy for euthanasia, but who also largely agreed that an enlightened, scientific, humane, and progressive society should legalize mercy killing, just as it should decriminalize birth control, enact eugenic laws, promote sex education, teach evolutionary theory, and enforce a strict separation of church and state.

In the coming decades, some individuals would join the American euthanasia movement only to support a personal and voluntary right to die. But to many, the distinction between involuntary and voluntary euthanasia was incidental. They would join because they, like Haiselden, saw euthanasia as a critical component of a broad reform agenda designed to emancipate American society from anachronistic and ultimately unhealthy ideas about sex, birth, and death. Details such as what constituted consent, and which lives were no longer worthy of life, rarely bothered Haiselden and his defenders. If his eugenic characterization of euthanasia was persuasive, it was not so much because it defined euthanasia merely in terms of eugenic theory, but because it conveyed the general impression that mercy killing was a cutting-edge reform congruent with the progress of science and modern secular values. This justification of euthanasia, powerfully attractive to Progressives, would outlast the Progressive era and continue to move the minds and hearts of Americans, until a cultural climate more critical of science and technology and paternalistic reform would materialize in the 1960s.

VI.

By 1917, and America's entry into World War I, Haiselden and euthanasia were vanishing from the nation's headlines. In July 1917 he allowed another newborn to expire, but war news quickly bumped him from the front pages. Mrs. Bollinger died that same month, brokenhearted, according to her husband, over the fateful decision she had made two years earlier. In the meantime, national attention shifted to other matters, such as the conflict overseas, the Armistice, the League of Nations, race riots, and the postwar "red scare" over communism. In 1919 Haiselden died in Cuba, where he had been conducting research in genetics and ways to improve the human race, a eugenicist to the last. By then he had been largely forgotten by the same public that only a few years earlier seemingly had followed his every move.

In a day and age when modern polling methods were unknown, it is impossible to tell whether popular support for euthanasia grew appreciably because of Haiselden's efforts, but with the debate over euthanasia tailing off in the 1920s, the likelihood is it did not. Euthanasia remained illegal and censured by the majority of Americans. Radical ideas such as a personal "right to cease to live" were anathema to a society, which, after World War I and especially in the midst of economic prosperity, was in no mood for groundbreaking reform that challenged traditional morals. The eugenic supporters of euthanasia tended to backtrack from making links between the two issues, shifting their energies instead to the campaign to enact immigration and eugenic sterilization laws, measures that seemed more in tune with the temper of the times. Euthanasia would attract a new crop of defenders in the 1930s when the climate for reform, radicalized by the sense of emergency produced by the Depression's economic devastation, proved more congenial to what President Franklin D. Roosevelt called "bold, persistent experimentation."[112]

Thus, the 1920s proved to be only a temporary lull in the history of the euthanasia movement. A crisis in mainstream Protestant churches in the 1920s would spawn liberal trends and encourage various reform-minded Americans involved in the campaigns for eugenics, female suffrage, socialized medicine, world peace, and birth control to question their faith and flock to the euthanasia colors in the 1930s. The debate over euthanasia would reignite over a series of highly publicized suicides in the thirties and the founding of the Euthanasia Society of America in 1938, providing momentum that helped to sustain the fledgling movement in the teeth of sometimes fierce opposition through to the 1960s. By then, changes in American society had revolutionized the entire euthanasia movement and transformed an old dispute into a modern-day culture war.

2

Breakthrough, 1920–1940

By the 1920s, euthanasia was no longer a secret in America. The popular and medical press had run stories on mercy killing, the first signs of a debate that would mark much of American life for the rest of the century. A motion picture, titled *The Black Stork,* about withholding surgery from a deformed newborn, had been released and was being shown commercially throughout the country. Clarence Darrow, Jack London, Eugene Debs, Helen Keller, and the editorial board of the *New Republic* had spoken out in favor of euthanasia.

Popular attitudes toward euthanasia also showed signs of movement. Most Americans in the interwar period agreed that there was something morally wrong about euthanasia as official policy, but that majority was growing slimmer as time went on. By 1939 roughly 40 percent of all Americans polled said they supported legalizing government-supervised mercy killing of the terminally ill. The times looked ripe for someone to exploit these shifts in popular sentiments.[1]

No one believed more adamantly that this moment had arrived

than the clergyman Charles Francis Potter, *the* central public figure within the American euthanasia movement during the first half of the twentieth century. Potter was an excellent example of the kind of person attracted to the euthanasia crusade in its early years. He was a tireless opponent of traditional religious doctrine and many of the inherited moral values that dominated American society and culture, as well as an advocate of eugenics, social Darwinism, and the mercy killing of severely handicapped inmates of state institutions.[2] Affable but argumentative, a witty champion of personal freedom yet sourly intolerant of opinions with which he disagreed, a seeming model of sincerity and a consummate actor, a defender of both individual choice and coercive social engineering—Potter was all these things and more. As such, he embodied perhaps more than any person the humane and paternalist motives existing in tense equilibrium within the euthanasia movement throughout much of the twentieth century. To Potter, any difficulties that might arise from trying to reconcile authoritarianism and the demands of humanity were amply overshadowed by an abiding and unquestioning progressivist faith in the power of science, medicine, and technology to liberate human beings from injustice and suffering. Utterly convinced that his cause was just, he believed the legalization of euthanasia would be the crowning glory to a life already dedicated to eugenics, birth control, world peace, the emancipation of women, and the defeat of Christian fundamentalism. When he died in 1962 just short of his seventy-seventh birthday, one of his few regrets was that he had not lived to see his hopes for euthanasia realized.

I.

The dispute over mercy killing, after subsiding in the 1920s, caught fire again in the 1930s, making these years a pivotal juncture in the history of euthanasia in America. With the coming of the Depression and more troubled economic times, Americans began talking again about suicide and controlled dying. Discussion of involuntary eugenic euthanasia also revived, despite the fact that during the 1930s support for eugenics among scientists was on the wane. Public opinion polls indicated in 1937 that fully 45 percent of Americans had caught up with Harry Haiselden's belief that the mercy killing of "infants born permanently deformed or mentally handicapped" was permissible.[3] Within the tense cultural atmosphere of the 1930s,

when grim economic conditions encouraged unconventional thinking on myriad social issues, euthanasia advocates enjoyed a receptive
climate for the first time since the heyday of Progressivism in the
early twentieth century. Led by people such as Charles Potter, they
went on the offensive, pressing the case for the legalization of mercy
killing. Without the coming of World War II and the publicity surrounding the horrors of Nazi mass murder, Potter's dreams of decriminalizing active euthanasia may well have been fulfilled within
his lifetime.

The euthanasia movement received invaluable publicity from the
frequent press reports of mercy-killing trials during the 1930s. These
cases often featured desperate parents killing their handicapped
children, or spouses putting their chronically ill loved ones to death.
Some defendants were acquitted, some given prison sentences, and
others committed to mental hospitals. In most instances, there was
no clear evidence that the victims had requested euthanasia formally. In other instances, individuals wracked with pain begged to
be put out of their misery. One woman in Buffalo, New York, severely injured in a car accident, told *Time* magazine in 1935 that she
wanted to die. "In the name of mercy, I ask you to appoint a doctor
to take my life," she pleaded with the Erie County Medical Association. Her words and those of others in similar circumstances helped
to personalize the right-to-die issue, prompting some Americans to
question their reflexive opposition to euthanasia.[4]

Just as a putative rise in the suicide rate sparked discussions of
euthanasia in the 1910s, so the perception that the United States
had plunged into a "suicide crisis" during the Depression caused
some Americans to express their toleration of euthanasia. The reported rate of people killing themselves went from 13.9 per 100,000
in 1929 to 17.4 in 1932. The suicide rate then leveled off in the mid-
1930s, possibly because those who had survived the initial years of
the Depression learned to adapt to the trying economic conditions.
Nonetheless, press coverage of the rise in the suicide rate was intense, feeding popular interest in the suicides of well-known figures.[5]

Two prominent Americans who took their own lives were George
Eastman and Charlotte Perkins Gilman. Eastman, founder of Eastman Kodak, ended his life in 1932 in his Rochester, New York, home
after a lengthy illness. Depressed from watching a close friend experience a protracted death, Eastman wrote a short note, asking
rhetorically: "My work is done. Why wait?" He then pointed a re-

volver at his heart and fired. Eastman's actions drew the sympathy of other well-known Americans, including the poet Carl Sandburg.[6]

Another high-profile suicide, occurring three years later, triggered considerable public debate. On 17 August 1935, the feminist Charlotte Perkins Gilman killed herself with chloroform in her Pasadena, California, home. Gilman was suffering from cancer, and rather than endure a prolonged and likely painful death, she decided to take her own life. Before doing so she, like Eastman, left a note, outlining her motives and stating how she "preferred chloroform to cancer." She also left with her literary agent an essay that was subsequently published. Typical of most Progressive defenders of euthanasia, Gilman not only endorsed the individual's right to choose the time, place, and means of death but also the community's right to perform "social surgery" by mercy killing persons who were no longer useful to fellow human beings. She lamented the "dragging weight of the grossly unfit" and urged their liquidation in the interests of "the normal and progressive."[7]

While one Catholic physician predictably condemned her actions, many other Americans agreed with Gilman, including suffragettes Carrie Chapman Catt and Harriet Stanton Blatch. They both thought her justified in taking her own life. These events surrounding Gilman's suicide were some of the first examples of a trend that would crystallize with more clarity in later years, that is, the historical affinity between supporters of euthanasia and the various reform movements dedicated to the emancipation of women.[8]

The novelist Sherwood Anderson also backed Gilman's behavior, as did the physician and sexologist Abraham Wolbarst. They agreed that society had a right to kill defectives whose lives consumed the community's resources. Anderson's and Wolbarst's comments were significant, since in a few short years they would become members of the Euthanasia Society of America.[9]

Wolbarst's remarks were a reminder that in the 1930s eugenics and euthanasia were still viewed as kindred causes by numerous social reformers, despite mounting scientific opposition to eugenics. As the decade wore on, more and more researchers and clinicians complained that eugenics was being exploited to justify racist and nativist sentiments. A consensus started to form that while the theory behind eugenics itself was not altogether wrong, its hereditarian basis was shaky. Geneticists argued that there were no single-unit hereditary characters for traits such as alcoholism, crime, or mental retardation. Thus, state eugenic sterilization laws would be ineffective in reducing the incidence of these conditions. Following the lead of Franz Boas, anthropologists contended that culture and environment were at least as powerful as instinct, biology, and nature in accounting for differences among human groups.[10]

However, some scientists, physicians, and social reformers refused to give up their allegiances to eugenics. The 1920s had been the highpoint of the eugenics movement, with many states passing sterilization laws, most of them compulsory in nature. From 1905 to 1922 eugenic sterilization laws were eventually enacted in fifteen states, but between 1923 and 1931 the number rose to twenty-eight. The 1927 U.S. Supreme Court ruling *Buck v. Bell* reassured eugenicists that sterilization laws would survive constitutional challenges, and some carried the campaign to other states in the 1930s.[11]

At the same time, many eugenicists felt that the next important crusade was to enact euthanasia laws. Invoking the eugenic language of another era, they repeated earlier calls for the use of a "lethal chamber" for painlessly disposing of defectives in the same way animals were put to death.[12] In 1931, the Illinois Homeopathic Medical Association defended euthanasia for "imbeciles and sufferers from incurable diseases."[13] Earnest Hooton, professor of anthropology at Harvard, similarly used social Darwinist reasoning to argue that euthanasia for "the hopelessly diseased and the congenitally deformed and deficient" was, like sterilization, absolutely necessary if America wished to reverse its ostensible biological decline.[14] His colleague at Harvard, professor of neurology William G. Lennox, agreed that euthanasia for society's "unproductive members" was warranted, although he stressed economic reasons. Other commentators claimed that the "time may come when it will be necessary to resort to euthanasia" for the eugenically unfit. These opinions were minority views, but, by the late 1930s, Americans were becoming more and more willing to conceive of euthanasia as a biologically as well as economically sensible policy.[15]

While Gilman, Wolbarst, Hooton, and Lennox all helped to sustain the debate over mercy killing in the 1930s, no one was more instrumental than Charles Francis Potter in making America "euthanasia-conscious."[16] As late as 1924, Potter had actually been opposed to euthanasia and did not openly endorse it until 1936. Yet, as he admitted later, his thinking had been headed in that direction for years. Born in 1885 in Marlboro, Massachusetts, Potter grew up in a strict Baptist family and in 1908 was ordained as a Baptist minister. However, even during these years, he was moving gradually away from the evangelical Christianity and biblical fundamentalism in which he had been raised and toward a belief that the only thing that redeemed human beings was their own potential creative power.[17]

The first sign of rebellion occurred in 1913 when he became a Unitarian pastor, and over the next few years he preached in several parishes in Canada and the United States. In 1919 he moved to West Side Unitarian Church in New York City, where he stayed until 1925. Meanwhile, he was gaining a national reputation for controversy, due to his support for women's equality, the League of Nations, eugenic sterilization, birth control, and the abolition of capital punishment. He also denounced the enforcement of the "blue laws" prohibiting people from work, shopping, and recreation on Sundays, praised secular rather than religious education, and asserted that science—especially Darwinist biology—trumped all religious doctrines.[18]

Potter burst onto the national scene in the 1920s, a crucial time in the history of religion in America. Protestant Christianity in the twenties was rocked by the rise of fundamentalism, defined as a belief in the accuracy and divine inspiration of scripture, the virgin birth of Christ, salvation solely through Christ's death on the cross, the bodily resurrection of Christ and his followers, and the authenticity of biblical miracles. None of these beliefs was new to American Christians by the turn of the twentieth century, but what made the fundamentalists different was their willingness to engage in public policy debates.[19]

The militant spirit of the fundamentalists derived from their perception that the beliefs they embraced were under attack from secular humanists. Fundamentalism, a term first coined in 1919, arose largely as a response to the development of evolutionary theory and literary higher criticism in the social sciences, both of which led liberal "modernist" Christians to question the infallibility and historical reality of scripture. Liberal modernists believed Protestant Christianity needed to assimilate these new trends in scholarship or Christianity might lose all credibility. Fundamentalists disagreed, arguing that modernism was both symptom and cause of a deeper crisis in postwar America, reflected in the horrors of the Great War, the unstable postwar peace settlement, the spread of labor unrest, and the specter of Bolshevik Communism dawning in eastern Europe.[20]

The rise of fundamentalism could not have come at a worse time for liberal modernist Christians, many of whom were undergoing a crisis of their own in the 1920s. Before World War I, most modernists had shared a fairly optimistic belief that science and progress were symbiotic. Modernists stressed the contingency and uncertainty surrounding events in natural and human history, but that did not shake their confidence that evolution was leading to higher levels of biological and social organization. Science—especially Darwinist biology—would provide human beings with new insights that society could use to manage and control nature for the benefit of the entire human race. Yet by the 1920s, the full implications of pragmatism, genetics, anthropology, paleontology, evolutionary naturalism, and Freudian psychology were beginning to sink in. Freud's pessimism about the ability of rational thought to control the mind's primitive drives appeared to describe to a tee a world just emerging from the savagery of world war and entering a period of radical political experiments. The rediscovery in the early twentieth century of Gregor Mendel's studies of inheritance in pea plants, by discrediting Darwin's own simplistic theories of heredity and variation, cast doubt on the notion of inevitable progress. The heyday of eugenics in the 1920s coincided with the growing sense that Darwin's fears about the degeneration of civilization were grounded in reality. Evolution, it seemed, could just as easily go backward as forward.[21]

The pragmatism of William James and Charles S. Pierce had similarly unsettling implications for the modernists. Pragmatists taught that truth varied from individual to individual and could be best judged according to its practical effects. As social scientists digested these ideas in the postwar years and questioned whether there were any absolute truths, faith in permanent values started to falter. Some American social scientists actually found these troubling thoughts to be quite bracing.[22] Harry Elmer Barnes, a future member of the ESA and close friend of Charles Potter, asserted in his controversial *The Twilight of Christianity* (1929) that the progress of modern knowledge had "spelled the doom of orthodox religion of any type whatsoever." Blaming religion for virtually all the unhappiness, injustice, ignorance, and suffering in the world, Barnes made it clear that only a revolutionary approach to ethics and morals could begin the process of reforming the world. "There was no reason to believe that social control based upon scientific knowledge cannot be made to pervade every aspect of human behavior," he wrote. Yet it was difficult to miss the hints of anxiety when he predicted that, were this project not realized, the result would be "chaos." Even someone so slavish to science feared that America had reached a crossroads fraught with dangers.[23]

The liberal modernist Christian minister Harry Emerson Fosdick, like Barnes a future ESA member, also believed that progress was not inevitable. Trying desperately to synthesize Christianity and the latest science, Fosdick argued in *Christianity and Progress* (1922) that Americans' faith in progress had made them complacent and created "a superficial, ill-considered optimism" that acted on the mind like an "opiate." "Social palliatives," based on this brand of optimism, would no longer be enough to "rescue" America; "radical cures" for the country's "public maladies" were necessary. Fosdick and Barnes did not agree on everything, but their common willingness to jettison much of orthodox religious teaching prepared them for their later conversion to the euthanasia cause.[24]

With both fundamentalists and modernists convinced that America had reached a perilous crossroads, conflict over who would determine the future was bound to be testy. At the center of the battle between fundamentalists and modernists was the theory of evolution and whether it should be taught. Fundamentalists cited the example of German militarism as a warning to Americans of where modernist adulation of science led. To explain German imperialist aggression, they readily pointed out how social Darwinism and the new biblical criticism had flourished in German schools before 1914. Therefore, the battle line for fundamentalists was drawn in the classroom, and their weapon of cultural war were state statutes outlawing the teaching of evolution.

No one welcomed this war more than the gadfly Potter. State laws prohibiting the teaching of evolution were an affront to everything he devoutly believed. To him, evolution not only *needed* to be taught in public schools; it had to be taught *instead of* religion.

The combination of Potter's feisty scientism and the growing militancy of fundamentalists led in 1923–24 to the highly publicized debates at Carnegie Hall between Potter and John Roach Straton, pastor of the Calvary Baptist Church in New York City. The twenties were a time of high interest in formal debates between opponents and defenders of evolutionary theory, and the Potter-Straton clash, broadcast live on radio, proved to be an entertaining show. Proclaiming that Americans faced a "crisis in theology" and only scientists ("the prophets of today") could solve it, the small, stocky, slightly balding Potter hammered away at literal interpretations of the Scriptures by invoking the theory of evolution and its ability to explain the origin of species and natural history. To the then-Unitarian Potter, Jesus Christ was not divine but simply an inspired reformer and moral teacher whose code of ethics should guide human conduct. It was precisely what this code of ethics stipulated that divided Straton and Potter.

The fundamentalist Straton won the debate with Potter on technical merit, but news of his bouts with Straton led the next year to Potter being invited to serve as religious adviser to lawyer Clarence Darrow at the Scopes "Monkey" trial in Dayton, Tennessee, from 1 July to 21 July 1925. Potter was only too happy to oblige.[25]

Potter's secular interpretations of religion made him a natural ally of the defense team surrounding teacher John Scopes, a group that included officials from the American Civil Liberties Union (ACLU) intent on testing in court Tennessee's 1925 statute prohibiting the teaching of evolution theory in public schools. Scopes, a high school biology teacher and part-time football coach, volunteered to serve as defendant, and was duly charged with violating the Tennessee law.

The Scopes trial, later immortalized in the play and movie *Inherit the Wind*, quickly became a media event, featuring a courtroom showdown between Darrow and the "Great Commoner" William Jennings Bryan, the thrice-defeated Democratic candidate for the U.S. presidency. By the 1920s, Bryan was a leading crusader against the teaching of evolution and eugenics. When the trial ended on 21 July 1925 Scopes was convicted and fined, but Bryan's death only days after a tense cross-examination at Darrow's hands in a sweltering courtroom left the impression that Bryan's defense of biblical fundamentalism had gone down to defeat. Appearances were deceptive, however. The fundamentalist crusade rolled on after the trial, so that by 1929 six other states had passed anti-evolution laws. Tennessee's own statute would not be repealed until 1967.[26]

Potter may have played an important role for Scopes's defense team behind the scenes, but publicly he was as much a liability as an asset. By this point in his life, Potter was denying the Bible contained divine wisdom, saying that it merely reflected an early stage of religious consciousness that by the twentieth century retained only Christ's moral teaching. He even dissented from the defense's public position that scripture and the theory of evolution were compatible. To Potter, evolution invalidated just about everything in scripture and orthodox theology and offered a handy rhetorical way of smearing opponents. "The author of the anti-evolution bill [in Tennessee] is obviously nearer in mental development to the nomads of early biblical times," Potter told the press, "than he is to the intelligence of the young man who is under trial." In Potter's eyes, orthodox Christians who disagreed with him were not just misinformed; they were in fact atavistic relics of a bygone era in the history of the human race, doomed to extinction through the blindly ruthless process of natural selection.[27]

In view of these opinions, Scopes's defense team understandably did not call Potter as an expert witness for the defense. As the journalist H. L. Mencken noted: "There is a Unitarian clergyman here from New York trying desperately to horn into the trial. He will fail. If Darrow ventured to put him on the stand the whole audience, led by the jury, would leap out of the courthouse windows, and take to the hills."[28] Potter had to content himself with giving the opening prayer at trial one day. Never one to pass up an opportunity to score a propagandistic point, he referred to God as merely "Thou to Whom all pray and for Whom are many names."[29]

The Scopes trial, far from being the consummation of Potter's career, turned out to be just another dramatic step closer to his open advocacy of euthanasia. Dissatisfied with the restraints on his freedom of expression in the pulpit at even ultraliberal Unitarian churches, in 1929 he resigned for good from any semblance of Christian preaching and founded the First Humanist Society of New York, a landmark event in the history of American religion and the nation's euthanasia movement. The First Humanist Society of New York in 1929 included as members John Dewey, Albert Einstein, Julian Huxley, Thomas Mann, George W. Rappleyea (of the John Scopes defense team), and Robert G. Ingersoll's granddaughter Eva Ingersoll Wakefield. The First Humanist Society, Potter boasted, had no creed, clergy, baptism, or prayer.[30]

Largely the brainchild of Potter and two other theologians, Curtis W. Reese and John H. Dietrich, Humanism emerged in the first three decades of the twentieth century as a type of religion heavily indebted to Unitarianism and liberal modernist Protestantism. Indeed, Potter, Dietrich, and Reese had all been Unitarians at one time. They brought with them Unitarianism's distinct fondness for interwar liberal causes, such as improved race relations, government economic planning, opposition to loyalty oaths, support for organized labor, the League of Nations, and world peace.[31]

Humanism, harking back to Robert Ingersoll's ideas, was Unitarianism's "most vital and distinctive theological movement since Transcendentalism." Humanism followed liberal Unitarian trends that not only denied the divinity of Christ but also questioned the supernatural and transcendental nature of God. As various liberal Unitarians contended in the early twentieth century, if God could be thought of as "that Love with which our souls commune," then God might simply be a symbol or name for the religious sentiment felt by most people. If so, then this religious sensibility was really an expression of the human personality itself. God had nothing to do with it, except insofar as God was the label people used to describe spiritual longing.[32]

Humanism's rejection of theism opened the door to a form of naturalist religion that was centered exclusively in humanity itself and borrowed liberally from developments in science. "Faith in man, that is my creed. . . . And that, my friends, is the very core of the new religion called Humanism," Potter told a radio audience in 1933.[33] That same year, Potter, along with thirty-three other intellectuals, signed the "Humanist Manifesto," containing the propositions that defined Humanism for Potter. The link between Unitarianism and the new Humanism was underscored by the fact that by the end of 1933 sixty Unitarian ministers had signed it. Humanism, according to the Manifesto, was a purely naturalistic religion, defined as "those actions, purposes, and experiences which are humanly significant." Religion is human life, and the goal of every human life is "the complete realization of the human personality."[34]

But how is the human personality realized to its fullest? Humanists, like classical nineteenth-century liberals, stressed individualism and the necessity to liberate people from religious superstition through education, science, medicine, and technology. However, Humanists did not approve of classical liberalism's vision of a society made up of rational, freely choosing, rugged individuals pursuing their own enlightened self-interest. As historian Perry Miller asked in 1942, "after [Unitarianism] had made men free to choose, what did it leave for them to choose?"[35] To Humanists, what redeemed the individual quest for personal realization was not the mere act of choosing but the causes individuals chose to support. In fact, it was through the very process of commitment and loyalty to worthwhile social causes that true freedom and personal fulfillment could be achieved. And what were these worthwhile causes? To Humanists, they were democracy, world peace, and the emancipation of individuals from the putative fatalism, prejudice, and ignorance of traditional religion. One was only free, then, when one subscribed to these anointed causes. Choosing not to was not a rational option; it was a negation of genuine freedom.

Little wonder, then, that Potter saw euthanasia as a quintessentially Humanist cause. For him, there was a logical sequence linking the time he became a Unitarian in 1913 and 2 February 1936 when he announced his support for legalized euthanasia before the First Humanist Society of New York. The influence of Humanism and his experience as a "marryin' and buryin' parson" had changed his mind by the 1930s. Claiming he had seen too many incurably ill parishioners die in agony and heard too many plead with him to be put out of their misery, Potter began touting mercy killing as humane and an example of individuals exercising control over their own destinies, a final, defiant "triumph over the flesh." He utterly rejected the orthodox Christian notion that God willed the suffering of terminally ill patients for the benefit of their souls. After all, he reasoned, organized medicine had overcome religious scruples in the past when it introduced anesthesia for surgery and used the science of bacteriology to fight infectious diseases. Why did either organized religion or medicine balk at euthanasia if mercy killing, when "legalized, safeguarded, and supervised by the state," held out the hope of reducing the painful torment of a patient's final hours? To Potter, dying was a life experience at least as significant as sex and reproduction. If women deserved the freedom to control their fertility through contraception, why did human beings not deserve the freedom to decide when, where, and how they died? Prohibiting this form of freedom was tantamount to stifling the development of an individual's creative personality. Where was "the spiritual value," he asked, "[w]hen men and women, in their final days of agony, damn their relatives and friends for permitting them thus to suffer, and even call down curses on the Almighty[?]"[36]

Besides, Potter asserted, what he called "bootleg euthanasia" was already happening. "For every mercy death you hear about there are ten you don't hear about." Physicians were secretly helping patients with incurable, painful diseases to die, and—Haiselden-like—were "putting out of misery malformed babies and idiot children whose lives mean nothing to themselves and whose existence is an ever-present nightmare to their parents." Using a rationale for euthanasia that would be cited frequently in the coming years, Potter recommended that euthanasia be legalized. Only that way could the usual "bungling amateur jobs" of nonphysicians be eliminated and potential abuses involving doctors and insensitive relatives be curtailed.[37]

As these comments indicated, Potter's support for euthanasia did not stop at voluntary mercy killing. Euthanasia was a worthy reform not just because it served humane, individual objectives and empowered people; it also served social purposes. For example, Potter argued in 1935, handicapped infants and the incurably insane and mentally retarded ought to be "mercifully executed by [the] lethal chamber."[38] "It is simply our social cowardice that keeps [imbeciles and idiot infants and 'monsters'] alive," he contended; their deaths were "socially desirable." The savings to a state such as New York would be enormous, something like $30 million. Recalling Harry Haiselden's rhetoric, Potter maintained that euthanasia also made eugenic sense, in that it prevented defectives from growing up and reproducing. As was the case with voluntary euthanasia, Potter recommended safeguards, including legal and medical permission and a waiting period. Yet there was no mistaking his opinion that euthanasia was a tax-saving, utilitarian, and biologically necessary public policy.[39]

Potter's belief that euthanasia and his Unitarian-inspired Humanism were philosophically linked was reflected in the fact that, among the leading figures of the euthanasia movement, there was an uncommonly large number of Unitarians and Humanists—surprising given their tiny representation in the American population. By emphasizing the obligation of responsible human beings to make specific life-affirming choices, Humanists such as Potter were entitled to think that euthanasia could be extended to include nonconsenting individuals. Freedom did not mean the license to do as one pleased. As he wrote in 1950, for social progress to occur "man must learn to play the game with more team spirit. Social responsibility is the lesson he must learn. The era of personal liberty had its attractions and the subordination of personal liberty to social progress is difficult but increasingly necessary." Evoking the positivist dream of Auguste Comte, Potter foresaw a world led by "sociopolitical engineers" who would need "a pretty complete knowledge of the principles of eugenics, including the values and dangers of contraception, sterilization, and other methods of regulating the number and quality of births." It was to these "engineers" that individuals, normal or subnormal, would have to "subordinate" their personal liberties. So confident was Potter in these "principles" that he remained untroubled by any potential for abuse. For him the risk of abuse was negligible in contrast to the enormous benefits the decriminalization of euthanasia would confer on humanity. Achieving the freedom to commit euthanasia, in short, would be the triumphant capstone to his entire career as preacher and social conscience of the nation.[40]

II.

Potter's views about euthanasia, nourished by Unitarianism, Humanism, and liberal modernism, dovetailed with those of several other American social reformers in the 1930s. While he was making headlines in New York, with less fanfare Inez Celia Philbrick, a Lincoln, Nebraska, physician and faculty member of the University of Nebraska, was in the process of trying to mobilize support for the country's first state euthanasia bill since the abortive Ohio initiative in 1906. Although her efforts in Nebraska did not succeed, no one— not even the better-known Potter—tried harder than Philbrick to advance the cause of euthanasia in twentieth-century America.

Philbrick was a woman with firm opinions about matters both great and small. As a teacher of home economics at the University of Nebraska, she endorsed midwifery, rejected pasteurization of milk, condemned competitive sports, denounced high heels for women, discouraged slim female figures as bad for childbirth, and advised all her women students to refrain from kissing their boyfriends until they were engaged.[41] A Unitarian, she supported women's suffrage, birth control, eugenic sterilization, world peace, and an end to child labor. She too criticized Christian fundamentalists for their faith in an inerrant Bible, especially their literal reading of the injunction "Thou shall not kill." To Philbrick, the commandment really meant "thou shall not commit murder," which she distinguished from mercy killing. She was one of the many defenders of euthanasia who in the twentieth century would use this interpretation of the commandment to deny there was any incompatibility between euthanasia and traditional religious teaching.

Philbrick also vilified Catholics who, like the National Catholic Women's Union (NCWU), justified physical suffering as a "blessing in disguise." Does the NCWU, she asked facetiously in 1947, "regard the thousands of men, women, and children in Spain living in utter degradation—cold, hungry, starving, diseased and tortured in Franco's detention camps—as recipients of blessing from church and state, rather than as victims of man's inhumanity?" Echoing the fierce anti-Catholicism that gripped the eugenics, euthanasia, and birth control movements during these years, Philbrick attacked the Church's opposition to contraception, accusing the Vatican of promoting poverty, disease, crime, and "births doomed inevitably to hereditary handicaps," such as mental retardation.[42]

Just as Potter had first-hand experience ministering to the dying, so Philbrick was aware of the suffering they all too often endured. In 1936 she lost a close friend to cancer. Her friend had spent her last six months of life bedridden and in excruciating pain that medication could not erase, but, fearing prosecution, she would not let Philbrick give her a lethal dose. Shortly after her demise, Philbrick decided to work for the legalization of active euthanasia.

Obviously, watching her friend slowly die was a catalytic personal experience for Philbrick, convincing her of the need for legalized euthanasia. Numerous others have joined the euthanasia movement because of similar experiences. Yet as important as the experience was, it does not explain why others who have witnessed similar heart-wrenching sights did not embrace euthanasia as a social reform. Nor does it explain why Philbrick refused to restrict euthanasia to only consenting and competent adults. Philbrick's decision to lobby for euthanasia legislation fit closely her general approach to social health and welfare as a feminist and maverick physician. Having defied convention for so long, she had developed the iconoclast's deep-seated faith in her own opinions. She personified the devoted country doctor, having delivered 2,100 babies in forty-two years of family practice, often under trying conditions. The story was told how once Philbrick had braved floods to deliver a baby for a woman whose house was surrounded by water and whom other doctors refused to treat.[43] This kind of behavior, when added to her defense of charity clinics, midwifery, natural childbirth, and socialized medicine, solidified her pariah status within her profession and ultimately led to her quitting the American Medical Association after thirty years of practice, complaining of medicine's commercialism and opposition to reform. To Philbrick, professional medicine was as serious an obstacle to enlightened and humane health care as was organized religion. In its rigid adherence to the Hippocratic Oath, prohibiting doctors from administering lethal doses, medicine denied dying patients the relief from suffering they desperately sought, Philbrick argued. A colorful contrarian, Philbrick was naturally inclined to champion a cause such as euthanasia that was condemned by most doctors.

Her variety of early twentieth-century maternal feminism reinforced her adherence to coercive euthanasia and explained her similar enthusiasm for eugenics.[44] To Philbrick, euthanasia, eugenics, and birth control were equally women's issues. Darwinist evolutionary theory taught that women were "superior" to men because they, as the "bearers of children," used "sexual selection" to determine which males of the species possessed the greatest physical size, strength, and overall fitness. Women's "supreme function" as the guardians of the race, she argued in 1929, meant they carried the

> responsibility of seeing that no child is born with handicap, that motherhood be released from bondage, and made a function of freedom, choice, and beauty. Specifically, on women physicians devolves the responsibility of informing themselves as to right and harmless and to-be-sure methods of birth control, and of instructing their patients in their use. Upon women physicians especially rests the responsibility of bringing about sterilization of the unfit, which measure alone can save civilization from annihilation.[45]

These views informed Philbrick's attitude toward euthanasia. As guardians of the race, women also had a special interest in mercy killing. Not only was euthanasia sensible in cases such as her friend's, but Darwinist biology justified the involuntary euthanasia of deformed infants and the mentally and physically handicapped. As she wrote, besides being a "merciful" method, "[i]n its social application the purpose of euthanasia is to remove from society living creatures so monstrous, so deficient, so hopelessly insane that continued existence has for them no satisfactions and entails a heavy burden on society." Euthanasia was such an important public health reform, according to Philbrick, that she thought it should be funded out of state taxes.[46]

Philbrick and Potter, then, thought alike. Euthanasia—either elective or without consent—was a humane means of biological, social, and individual improvement, just like birth control. For the combative Philbrick, the struggle between organized religion and professional medicine over birth control seemed to be won with the 1936 *One Package* U.S. Appeals Court decision that permitted physicians to receive contraceptive information and devices in the mail. In her opinion, the war over euthanasia against the same foes was just beginning. She was not the only advocate of euthanasia in twentieth-century America to think this way.

Armed with these thoughts, in 1937 Philbrick sought to have a euthanasia bill introduced in the unicameral Nebraska legislature.[47] Legislative Bill No. 135, given Philbrick's pronounced opinions about eugenic euthanasia, was fairly moderate. The legislation made it possible for adults of "a sound mind" and suffering from "an incurable and fatal" illness to apply to a district judge for merciful death. The application would be forwarded to a committee of two doctors and one lawyer, and if all requirements had been met and the judge and committee approved, then the patient's attending physician could administer the lethal dose. Yet the bill also included provisions for "mental incompetents" and "minors" suffering from an incurable or fatal diseases, in which cases "next of kin" could apply on their behalf.[48]

Although the Nebraska bill contained clauses permitting involuntary euthanasia, Philbrick foresaw even broader legislation in the future. She believed that limiting the bill to patients suffering from "incurable and fatal" disease was unfair to the many consenting people who were not exactly dying but still had incurable illnesses or conditions (such as amyotrophic lateral sclerosis, or Lou Gehrig's disease). To Philbrick, they ought to have been eligible for euthanasia. As someone who favored existing eugenic sterilization laws, she also hoped that similar statutes would ultimately be passed legalizing the euthanasia of institutionalized mental patients and the mentally retarded. It was not enough to permit the euthanizing of these kinds of patients with the consent of their parents or guardians. A comprehensive euthanasia bill ought to be "mandatory," she wrote to Potter in late 1937, "in the case of idiots (living beings with whom communication is impossible), monstrosities, the insane, suffering from certain types of insanity, in which incurability has been established after a term of years during which there has been expert supervision and study." The "criminal insane," she added, "should always be put to death humanely." As someone who hated anything less than utter candor, Philbrick disliked watering down the Nebraska bill to make it more palatable to public opinion, but she recognized it was necessary until a future date when Americans were more used to the idea of some broader form of legal euthanasia.[49]

Philbrick may have thought that her Nebraska bill was sugar-coated, but to no one's surprise it never was considered in the state legislature.[50] The Nebraska State Medical Association, the University of Nebraska School of Pharmacy, the editor of the *Journal of the American Medical Association*, and most clergymen opposed the bill. As a physician herself who had fought the profession on other issues, Philbrick found the medical resistance particularly bothersome. As she put it, "it seems not to have occurred in the minds of many of the profession that the Oath of Hippocrates, dating from the fourth century B.C., . . . may need amendment to meet the thought and needs of the twentieth century A.D." The state medical association countered by claiming that the progress of medicine meant more and more illnesses were proving amenable to treatment and could not be defined as fatal, a point borne out in the 1940s with the introduction of penicillin and the discovery in 1947 of the Salk vaccine for polio.[51]

However, medical history was on Philbrick's side. America was in the midst of a major transition in public health. As the mortality rate of acute, infectious diseases declined during the twentieth century, life expectancy rose, and the major causes of death became chronic degenerative diseases, chiefly strokes and heart attacks, or neoplasms such as cancer and sarcomas. While medical science and technology became better able to keep chronically ill patients alive for longer periods than ever before, thanks to chemotherapy, artificial respiration, renal dialysis, and organ transplants, the age of the "magic bullet" was largely over by mid-century. These trends would culminate in a crisis for organized medicine by the 1970s, when growing numbers of Americans would face the haunting prospect of a long, drawn-out, and likely painful death. By then, Philbrick's views on euthanasia would look much less radical than they did in the 1930s.[52]

Characteristically, Philbrick was undaunted by her defeat in Nebraska. She took satisfaction in the fact that the proposed bill had attracted considerable press interest.[53] With her keen sense of the state's politics, Philbrick decided to leave the campaign for legalized euthanasia in the hands of allies and moved to Dayton, Ohio, where she thought a tougher euthanasia law stood a better chance of passing. Yet she proved no more successful in Ohio than she had been in Nebraska. Events occurring in Europe in the 1940s would deal her and the euthanasia movement a powerful blow.[54]

It is tempting to dismiss Philbrick as an extremist, but within the fledgling euthanasia movement she was far from exceptional. Many who gravitated to the movement in the 1930s shared her reasons for supporting euthanasia legislation. They could point to the several high-profile cases of suicide, like George Eastman's or Charlotte Perkins Gilman's, or press accounts of distraught relatives putting family members out of their misery. Yet humane reasons often coexisted with eugenic considerations and frequently in the same person's mind. Many early defenders of euthanasia, coming from the birth control and eugenics movements, cited social, biological, economic, or humanitarian justifications interchangeably, without apparently seeing any inconsistency. Some undoubtedly favored one rationale over another, yet, in the case of Potter and Philbrick—individuals with backgrounds in a variety of bona fide liberal and progressive causes—on close inspection these motives prove to be difficult to disentangle. Their neo-Progressive approaches to euthanasia were fundamentally linked to their broad ways of looking at the world, a world they saw in dire need of reform and enlightenment. And nothing more deserved reform than the legal circumstances surrounding death and dying. Only when the taboo against mercy killing was toppled could this type of reform begin in earnest.

III.

In the meantime, Potter's 1936 address on euthanasia had attracted others to the euthanasia standard, such as Mrs. R. L. (Ann) Mitchell, the cofounder, with Potter, of the Euthanasia Society of America. While individuals like Potter and Philbrick supplied the public relations and the political activism, Mitchell, more than anyone else, provided the much-needed cash to sustain the euthanasia movement in its first few difficult years.

Mitchell's unstable personality made her best suited to a behind-the-scenes role. A wealthy New Yorker, she had been hospitalized from 1934 to 1936 at the Bloomingdale asylum as a mental patient and was likely psychotic when, in 1942, she committed suicide by throwing herself out of a Miami, Florida, hotel window. Whether nature or nurture was more to blame for her emotional troubles is unclear. What is clear is that the failure of her family to share her enthusiasm for euthanasia led to considerable domestic friction—so bad that she divorced her husband and tried to disinherit her two sons just before she killed herself.

Mitchell's experience as an institutionalized mental patient profoundly shaped her views about euthanasia. She was convinced there was "a terrible strain of heredity" afflicting her and her extended family. This theory led her to conclude that all mental patients were helpless in the grip of a relentless genetic disease. To Mitchell, psychiatrists were of no use when it came to curing mental illness, and in most cases they did more harm than good for their patients. She concluded that the merciful, eugenic, and economically responsible thing to do was to legalize the mercy killing of such patients so they might "find peace . . . and not live in that intolerable hell that we lived in before, with the bars enclosing us in our torture and a nurse guarding us day and night so that we cannot escape to peace." In other words, Mitchell was less interested in voluntary, active euthanasia for rational adults than in nonelective mercy killing of mentally incompetent asylum patients and defective infants. She even believed endorsing a "monster birth bill" that covered euthanasia for severely handicapped babies would help to attract "younger women" to the movement. Support for involuntary mercy killing would turn out to be a fairly common attitude among early proponents of euthanasia, and, like later supporters of a right to die, much of Mitchell's fervor for euthanasia was due to her dim view of physicians' competence in healing the sick and dying.[55]

Mitchell may have been "crazy," as her husband alleged, but there is no discounting how instrumental she was in helping to found the ESA.[56] By 1936 she had become interested in euthanasia and had learned that a pro-euthanasia organization had been formed in England in December 1935, with headquarters in the city of Leicester. Called the Voluntary Euthanasia Legislation Society (VELS), it had been founded by C. Killick Millard, a retired public health physician from Leicester. Millard's career promoting euthanasia, although spent in England, featured many similarities linking euthanasia advocates on both sides of the Atlantic. A Unitarian like many supporters of euthanasia in America, he resembled other iconoclastic reformers interested in euthanasia. Besides rejecting compulsory infant vaccination for smallpox, Millard championed temperance, eugenics, cremation, and birth control. He was convinced that when public health was at stake, nothing was taboo.

His Leicester background was crucial in shaping these views. The city had a long and distinctive history of religious dissent and libertarianism, nonconformism, and radical politics stretching back to the early nineteenth century. Millard the Unitarian was thus doubly predisposed to reject the traditional Christian prohibition against ending one's own life, even in great pain and suffering. He breathed in Leicester's air in more than one respect, and only after his death in 1952 did the VELS shift its headquarters to London.[57]

Millard spent the years between 1931 and 1935 assembling an impressive group of English physicians, clerics, scientists, and writers—including Havelock Ellis, H. G. Wells, and Julian Huxley. As would be the case with the ESA, many of the inaugural members of the VELS were adherents to eugenics, including Millard himself.[58] In 1936, he managed to get a voluntary euthanasia bill introduced into Great Britain's House of Lords, but after some spirited debate a second reading was postponed for six months, a "polite way of moving the rejection of the bill," in Millard's own words. Millard and the VELS had never expected the bill to pass in the first place and were satisfied with the fact that the Lords debate had received considerable press coverage.[59]

Inspired by the VELS example, Mitchell sprang into action, contacting Potter about the possibility of setting up an American euthanasia organization with her financial assistance. Potter was keenly interested and began corresponding with leading American figures in the hopes of recruiting them. Potter's pitch stressed the humane, economic, and eugenic dimensions of euthanasia, a message that proved to have wide appeal within America's elite social, literary, and academic circles. Especially powerful was Potter's theory that euthanasia was consistent with Christian concepts of mercy. By late 1937 he, like Millard in England, had assembled a lengthy list of prominent individuals willing to join the new organization, including Robert Frost, Somerset Maugham, Sherwood Anderson, Fannie Hurst, Rex Stout, and Max Eastman. He was also able to recruit the well-known physician Walter Alvarez and physiologist Walter B. Cannon. On 16 January 1938 he announced the founding of the National Society for the Legalization of Euthanasia (NSLE), quickly renamed the Euthanasia Society of America (ESA).[60]

On paper the new ESA looked impressive, but like the VELS it was small and elitist. It numbered barely 200 members by the end of the 1930s, was led by a tiny, upper-class social circle located in Manhattan, and could not afford to keep an office open five days a week. Its ability to draw press attention and depict itself as a group defending popular sentiments and needs disguised the embarrassing fact that it was anything but a grassroots organization.

While Mitchell served as both ESA secretary and board member until her death in 1942, Potter withdrew from its presidency in December 1938, pleading that, because he had never received a salary and had to earn a living from lecturing and writing, he had little time to devote to the group's everyday operation. He also complained about neglecting his responsibilities to the Humanist Society, out of whose office he had managed the ESA. On the other hand, he believed he was leaving the ESA in good condition, claiming that the ESA had enjoyed "more progress in one year than the birth control movement did during its first 10 years."[61]

Officially, Potter vacated the ESA's presidency amicably, but it was also true that sparks had begun to fly between him and Mitchell. Shortly before she died, she accused him of being "absolutely dishonest and untrustworthy" and far more interested in money than the euthanasia cause. When Potter reputedly tried to get his son on the ESA payroll at $200 a week, it was the last straw for Mitchell.[62] Some of her charges were doubtless due to her increasingly delusional mental state, but it is significant that Philbrick and other women members of the ESA defended her. Some of Potter's difficulties with Mitchell undoubtedly were his own fault, and, as was the case in the birth control movement, tensions along gender lines were never far from the surface in the euthanasia movement. The male figures, who tended to be professionals, preferred to dictate policy and delegate the secretarial work to women. Such behavior was bound to annoy the women who made up more than half of the core group that attended early ESA meetings. To the women who had felt empowered by their participation in the struggle to improve women's health and separate sex from reproduction through the use of contraception, the presence of men such as Potter who monopolized the headlines and got most of the credit in the campaign for euthanasia was a source of frustration. So, too, were Potter's persistent claims right to the day he died that he alone had founded the ESA.[63]

Despite these signs of gender tension, the early membership of the ESA reflected the common way many educated men and women viewed euthanasia. Rather than defend it in the language of individual rights, members often perceived it as a eugenic matter, good for the interests of humanity and society in general. A striking 73 percent of the ESA's founders were supporters of eugenics.[64] By the early 1940s, the list of ESA advisory council members who had defended eugenics to one degree or another was long. Besides Philbrick and Potter, the list included notable Americans Margaret Sanger, the internationally renowned birth control activist; Lewellys F. Barker, the Johns Hopkins University internist; Leon F. Whitney, executive secretary of the American Eugenics Society from 1924 to 1934 and author of *The Case for Sterilization* (1934); journalist Albert Edward Wiggam, author of the *New Decalogue of Science* (1923) and member of the American Eugenics Society and Potter's First Humanist Society of New York; clergyman Harry Emerson Fosdick, member of the American Eugenics Society advisory council from 1923 to 1935; Henry H. Goddard, professor of psychology at Ohio State University; Foster Kennedy, professor of neurology at Cornell Medical College; Edward A. Ross, professor of sociology at the University of Wisconsin; Arthur A. Estabrook, biologist and member of the American Eugenics Society advisory council; William McDougall, professor of psychology at Duke University; George H. Parker, Harvard zoologist; Sidney E. Goldstein, Rabbi of the Free Synagogue of New York and supporter of the Ethical Culture Society; Samuel J. Holmes, University of California zoologist; and Harry Elmer Barnes, a member of the advisory board of Potter's First Humanist Society of New York. Among the eugenicist VELS members who also joined the newly formed ESA were C. Killick Millard, H. G. Wells, Havelock Ellis, and Julian Huxley.

Eugenicists similarly stood out on the ESA's executive and board of directors. Besides Potter, they included Clarence Cook Little, president of both the University of Michigan and the American Society for the Control of Cancer; Robert Latou Dickinson, noted gynecologist and birth control advocate; Oscar Riddle, researcher at the Carnegie Station of Experimental Evolution; Frank H. Hankins, sociologist at Clark University and Smith College; Stephen S. Visher,

Indiana University geographer; Walter F. Willcox, professor of economics and statistics at Cornell University; and Wyllistine Goodsell, professor of education at Columbia. Not all American eugenicists joined the ESA, nor were all ESA members eugenicists. Nor did all ESA eugenicists join the organization solely for eugenic reasons. Some ESA eugenicists such as Margaret Sanger and C. Killick Millard never went as far as Harry Haiselden in supporting euthanasia for eugenic reasons. Instead, they tended to view euthanasia in terms of society's obligation to provide all deserving Americans with the choice of a merciful death. The avid eugenicist Albert Wiggam lent his name to the ESA primarily because he was so distressed about the suffering his wife and brother endured when they died.

Nonetheless, the conspicuous representation of eugenicists in ESA ranks underlines the close kinship between the two issues in Depression-era America. While personal tragedies provided emotional motives for joining the ESA, adherence to eugenics helped to rationalize the rejection of traditional morality that paved the way for the acceptance of euthanasia. Eugenics, with its affinities to social Darwinism and scientific naturalism, convinced thinkers such as Wiggam that, when faced with difficult decisions about birth, sex, and death, the old gods were dead and the old rules no longer applied. A new set of values and a new code of ethical conduct were required to provide Americans with the policy choices they needed to adapt to the rapidly changing social conditions of twentieth-century life.[65]

Ann Mitchell was perhaps the most outspoken of all ESA members on the eugenic dimensions of euthanasia. In 1939 she welcomed the coming of World War II and hoped it would last "a long time," giving countries such as Britain and the United States an opportunity to do some serious "biological house cleaning." "We must breed human beings as carefully as we do animals," she wrote, urging "euthanasia as a war measure, including euthanasia for the insane, feeble-minded monstrosities." Such tactics were necessary, she continued, if the democracies wanted to defeat Nazi Germany. She believed wholeheartedly that the war was a life-or-death contest for biological supremacy that would be decided by the nations most willing to put euthanasia and eugenics into practice.

Due to Mitchell's pronounced opinions, the ESA executive understandably did its best to keep her away from the public spotlight as much as possible. Yet, as subsequent events would demonstrate, her opinions about the biological and social significance of euthanasia were not all that different from those of many of her colleagues at the ESA.[66]

IV.

The first priority of the new society, besides drawing up its bylaws and constitution, was to design a model euthanasia bill so local state groups could begin the process of introducing legislation. Since under the Constitution Congress had no power to legislate euthanasia, such change had to occur at the state level.[67] Most members of the ESA agreed that a euthanasia law should cover incurably ill people who voluntarily requested their doctors to put them out of their misery. The organization was heartened by a recent national poll that showed that as many as 64 percent of Americans in the Mountain and Pacific Coast regions endorsed elective physician-administered euthanasia. The consensus was that a law covering this form of euthanasia would only legalize the "bootleg euthanasia" physicians were already practicing. Using thinking that would later be exploited to justify decriminalizing abortion, Potter and others argued that there would be disrespect for the law if it said one thing and people did the exact opposite.[68]

The main thrust of the ESA's message in 1938 was that legalizing elective euthanasia for terminally ill patients, dying in agony from a disease such as cancer, was one of the most merciful and Christian things someone could do for another human being. Behind closed doors, however, with so many eugenicists on the ESA's board, it is hardly surprising that there was strong sentiment in favor of extending euthanasia to cover unconscious geriatric patients, the incurably insane, and handicapped infants and children. At the same time, board members were acutely aware that their chances of getting a state legislature to pass such a bill were almost nonexistent. In the case of insanity and mental retardation, more and more evidence was surfacing that various treatments could at least mitigate the severity of symptoms and improve the quality of patients' lives. Over Mitchell's objections, Wyllistine Goodsell cited the 1936 American Neurological Association report that questioned the hereditary basis of both psychosis and mental retardation. Goodsell had been trained by John Dewey as an educational psychologist. Besides belonging to the ESA and American Eugenics Society, she was also a member of the American Civil Liberties Union and a founder of the

Women's Faculty Club at Columbia University.[69] "There are certain children born congenital idiots and of course I don't think we should keep them alive at all," Goodsell remarked in 1938, but she believed it was too difficult to convince professionals and the American public to endorse such mercy killing without more hard evidence that congenital idiots were genetically doomed. Like others on the ESA board of directors, she felt it was important to "follow the line of least resistance," and first fashion a bill limited to euthanasia for consenting, chronically ill patients whose incurability was certified by a team of physicians.[70]

For the time being, then, tactics eclipsed principles. Board members agreed that "the immediate objective [was] to get a bill passed as an entering wedge," in Potter's words. "Later on we want to include certain types of insanity," he added. Or, as another member said: "Get a bill passed to allow that one thing [voluntary euthanasia] and it will be easier to get more in later." At its 30 March 1938 meeting, the ESA board decided to follow the example of the VELS and support only voluntary euthanasia. As events over the next half-century would prove, some ESA members continued to believe this resolution was only a temporary expedient.[71]

The ESA model euthanasia bill that emerged from these deliberations was, at least in the opinion of most ESA members, heavily safeguarded and eminently moderate. Someone who desired euthanasia had to be at least twenty-one years of age, "of sound mind," and "suffering from severe physical pain" caused by an incurable disease. The patient then had to petition a court in writing with the signatures of two witnesses and the attending physician, who would testify to the incurable nature of the illness and the competent mental state of the patient. Next, the court would appoint a committee of three members, two of whom had to be doctors, to examine the petition and its signatories. If at least two committee members approved the petition, a person selected by the patient could administer euthanasia. Significantly, to reassure anxious physicians, anyone who either performed or assisted the act of euthanasia would be immune from criminal or civil liability.[72]

Despite its many safeguards, no state politicians agreed to sponsor the bill, although a handful expressed sympathy with the ESA's efforts. Clearly, state legislators, no matter how they felt about euthanasia, believed that it was political suicide to support its legalization. This was especially true in states with sizable Catholic populations, such as New York, the main target of ESA efforts. Flexing the formidable political muscle Roman Catholicism enjoyed in 1930s America, Catholic organizations repeatedly condemned euthanasia and the ESA. As the president of Fordham University declared in 1939, "Western civilization hangs in the balance, and indifference on the part of society might cause its downfall. It is through indifference that conditions exist whereby doctors may advocate murder in the form of mercy-killing, ministers may preach for birth-control and divorce, and judges may accept graft and bribery." Politicians, conscious of the Catholic influence at the ballot box, paid careful heed to these kinds of Church statements.[73]

Protestant groups also expressed their fears that euthanasia would be abused if it were not prohibited by law. As was the case during the Bollinger controversy—and would be for decades to come—organized medicine likewise strongly opposed legalizing euthanasia. No matter how much the ESA tried to moderate its position on the legalization of euthanasia, it was obvious that the most powerful mainstream interest groups in America did not share its enthusiasm for the cause. Despite the suggestive findings of opinion polls in the late 1930s, the time simply was not ripe for such a legislative reform.

Another bone of contention for the fledgling ESA that would emerge again and again in later years was the choice of name for the new organization. Almost immediately the decision was made to replace the name National Society for the Legalization of Euthanasia with something more reflective of the organization's goals. The board settled on the Euthanasia Society of America at its 3 May 1938 meeting, thanks mainly to Rabbi Sidney Goldstein. Goldstein, born in 1879 in Marshall, Texas, and a professor of sociology at the Jewish Institute of Religion in New York City, was another example of the kind of liberal progressive drawn to the euthanasia movement. Besides support for eugenics, he was a firm defender of birth control, marriage counseling, organized labor, and international disarmament. An advocate of women's suffrage and a staunch opponent of patriarchy, he criticized husbands and fathers who did not involve their wives and children in family decision making. The only thing wrong with Roosevelt's New Deal, according to Goldstein, was that it did not go nearly far enough to provide work for the unemployed.[74]

Goldstein's vision for the ESA was not restricted to efforts at legalizing euthanasia. He wanted the ESA to engage in a major "educational program" to advance the general idea of euthanasia. He envisaged euthanasia as another issue synonymous with the progressive reform of society; acceptance of euthanasia would lead to the dismantling of barriers to personal emancipation in numerous other fields of human endeavor. Legalization, while important, was no more urgent than preparing Americans to exercise the personal autonomy that euthanasia dictated. Like Potter, he wanted the ESA to take the lead in such public education efforts. Like Potter, he also blurred the fine line between advocating choice and recommending euthanasia as an enlightened and rational solution to specific problems. As someone who viewed eugenics and euthanasia as kindred causes, Goldstein was as fervent a believer in an expansive definition of mercy killing as were most of his colleagues in the ESA.[75]

By criticizing the inclusion of the word "legalization" in the ESA's title, Goldstein was rehearsing the later (and often bitter) conflict within the euthanasia movement between members who wanted to devote their full energies to the enactment of euthanasia laws and those more interested in encouraging a wide public debate over death and dying. Defenders of keeping "legalization" in the name tended to feel that state legislatures were the front lines of the battle to win public approval of euthanasia. Once one state passed a bill, then other statutes would follow, including ones that permitted the mercy killing of incompetent children and adults. Legislative success would compel public opinion to accept euthanasia. Defenders of legalization also argued that if the word was good enough for the British VELS, why was it not good enough for its American counterpart? Goldstein and others dissented, favoring the ESA's educational function. As a result, the name Euthanasia Society of America remained unchanged over the next twenty-nine years. But the conflict between those within the ESA who preferred a policy of public education and those who wanted to dedicate themselves to legalizing euthanasia through the political process continued to simmer. By the 1970s this difference of opinion had grown so acrimonious it would split the euthanasia movement.

The decision to limit ESA official policy to support of voluntary euthanasia legislation proved difficult to enforce. Ann Mitchell was not the organization's only ticking public relations bomb. The neurologist Foster Kennedy, who succeeded Potter as ESA president in 1939, believed like Mitchell that the most urgent need was to legalize euthanasia for the severely mentally retarded—what he called "nature's mistakes"—and not for "normal adults, who having become ill, are going down into the shadows." As he told the New York press in 1939, death was not "all it's cracked up to be," nor was he "concerned with the bleatings about pain." It was only "absurd and misplaced sentimental kindness" that kept society from mercy killing "a person who is not a person."[76]

These statements alone were contentious enough. However, to the embarrassment of the ESA, Kennedy based his support of euthanasia for "nature's mistakes" rather than for competent adults on his belief that medical diagnosis of incurability was so often wrong. In 1942 he recounted one of many examples he claimed to have seen of patients diagnosed with cancer, a seventy-two-year-old woman given only six months to live by two of New York's finest doctors. After putting her affairs in order and departing for her country home to die, she lived for another five years. "I could add to this case scores of others," Kennedy stated; and "besides, a civilization that deliberately shuts itself off from the bearing of pain and the presence of struggle and finally makes its bid for the softer life or death, is already slipping down the ways."[77]

Although Kennedy made it clear he was speaking as a private citizen and not officially as ESA president, the damage was done. His remarks drew sharp rebukes from the press and other physicians, not the kind of attention the ESA wanted. Besides belying the ESA's stated policy of supporting only voluntary euthanasia, such publicity also called into question the organization's faith in doctors' ability to diagnose fatal illnesses. If physicians were often in error about prognosis and diagnosis, then legalizing a mercy-killing process based on such medical expertise was fraught with the potential for abuse.

Kennedy's lack of sympathy for consenting adults who choose suicide as a way of escaping pain also created problems for the ESA. Having announced that it would lobby only for voluntary euthanasia for dying patients, it now faced the spectacle of a prominent member of its executive condemning precisely this kind of practice.

Kennedy's short presidency, lasting less than two months in early 1939, reflected the fact that the ESA consisted of many independently minded individuals who had firm opinions about euthanasia and how to run a reform organization. Kennedy's presidency also revealed that the ESA could not afford such publicity as it struggled to avoid further controversy. Euthanasia as a reform was controversial enough. Due to its membership, the ESA already projected the image of an elitist organization bent on telling ordinary Americans what was best for them. Until belief in traditional mores started to decline, and until a greater percentage of Americans endured the kind of end-of-life experiences the ESA described in its literature, the chances of public sympathy swinging solidly behind the ESA were slim. Utterances such as Kennedy's did nothing to help the ESA move closer to this goal.[78]

V.

Nonetheless, by the outbreak of World War II, the ESA had some grounds for optimism. Foster Kennedy was succeeded by the esteemed and more polished Clarence Cook Little, whose experience as president of the American Society for the Control of Cancer would stand him in good stead over the next few rocky years. Many Americans approved of physicians putting patients with terminal illnesses or disabilities to death painlessly, even if they did not want the practice legalized. While the ESA had found no one in the New York State legislature willing to introduce its model euthanasia bill, its members could congratulate themselves on the formation of a society blessed with the patronage of a growing membership that included many well-known Americans. It was true that the ESA was strapped for funds and facilities and faced an uphill battle to win over the hearts and minds of Americans. Yet it did not underestimate its opposition and heavily counted on the persuasive powers of people such as Potter and Goldstein to change public opinion.

Thus, the ESA had good reason to believe that trends already in motion in American society and culture would ultimately carry it to victory. As one ESA member confided in 1939, the euthanasia movement "is in the first difficult years, where the birth control movement was twenty years ago and the woman suffrage movement fifty years ago."[79] Or, as the perennially optimistic Potter put it in 1940, euthanasia was "rapidly emerging from the stage when it was considered merely the obsession of a few left-wing social reformers to the period when it is being recognized as an important social measure in the same class with birth control and eugenics."[80] The victories of the eugenics, birth control, and women's suffrage campaigns gave the many members of the ESA who had fought those earlier battles reason to hope that similar triumphs were in store for the euthanasia movement. The taboos against birth control, eugenic sterilization, and the women's vote had just been toppled, and the taboo against euthanasia appeared to be next. People such as Potter were convinced that gradually all rational Americans would come around to seeing the issue through the eyes of Humanists, forcing organized medicine to "give its sanction to euthanasia," in Phil-brick's words.[81] Once that happened, the forces of orthodox Christianity too would retreat, freeing Americans from religious superstition and tyranny.

Unfortunately for the ESA, it was counting on the momentum of the 1930s to continue. However, history was about to take an abrupt turn, presenting the ESA with a challenge it likely never anticipated and certainly never welcomed. Over the next two decades the ESA's resources and determination would be severely taxed as it struggled to adapt to changing cultural, social, and political circumstances. Euthanasia advocates would have to wait until another twist in history—the cultural, political, and social ferment of the 1960s and 1970s—for their fortunes to revive.

3

Stalemate, 1940–1960

When the 1940s dawned, many in the euthanasia movement believed it was only a matter of time before euthanasia became
legal in the United States. The 1930s had been marked by a flurry
of encouraging events, from headline-grabbing mercy killings to the
founding of the Euthanasia Society of America and England's Voluntary Euthanasia Legislation Society.

But euthanasia advocates were in for a surprise. At the very time
they were lobbying to get a voluntary euthanasia bill introduced into
the New York State legislature, the ground beneath them began to
shift seismically. World War II broke out, and as Hitler's war machine
marched eastward across Europe in late 1939, news of Nazi atrocities
against mental patients and handicapped children filtered back to
America. Euthanasia defenders in the United States discovered to
their horror that many Americans associated their movement with
these murders. For a group that prided itself on its liberalism, humanitarianism, and progressive views, the stigma of Nazism was particularly embarrassing.

Initially caught off guard, euthanasia proponents in America over the balance of the century struggled mightily to avoid the taint of Nazism. At the same time, they faced a resurgent Roman Catholic Church that used its considerable cultural and political clout to attack not only euthanasia but eugenics and birth control as well. The good news for euthanasia advocates was that being caught up in this larger cultural war won them some high-profile allies. The adversity they experienced as a target of Catholic attacks also helped them maintain a veneer of unity that papered over their differences. The bad news was that entanglement in these debates over Catholic power damaged the euthanasia movement's efforts to appear mainstream and moderate. It was not until the 1960s, when euthanasia advocates adopted new policies and the nation's cultural and social climate underwent a sea change, that the movement's fortunes began to improve, a reminder of how embedded the fortunes of the right to die have been in the main currents of American history. But until then, the euthanasia movement would learn some hard lessons in public relations and power politics.

I.

At the same time as Charles Potter, Inez Philbrick, and the rest of the ESA were preaching the virtues of euthanasia to the American public, a handful of German bureaucrats were at work on a sinister project that, besides casting a long shadow over all of twentieth-century German medicine, would set the American euthanasia movement back years. These Nazi officials were organizing the murder of more than 200,000 inmates from mental hospitals, correctional institutions, and old-age homes throughout central and eastern Europe. Included in that number were also incapacitated concentration or slave labor camp prisoners. Victims were either shot, gassed, overdosed, starved to death, or dispatched by lethal injections, and then cremated in six designated killing centers around Germany.

To American euthanasia proponents, the news of these atrocities was a nightmare. As word spread in the late 1940s, the euthanasia movement found itself increasingly on the defensive, scrambling to deny that the form of euthanasia it supported was the same as Nazi murder. While advocates sincerely believed that their brand of euthanasia had nothing to do with Hitlerian medical killing, many Americans failed to recognize the difference.

Numerous German physicians, psychiatrists, nurses, civilians, soldiers, and bureaucrats participated in this program of medical murder, first code-named "Aktion T-4" after the street address of its office headquarters, Tiergartenstrasse 4. In August 1941 the Aktion T-4 program was closed down in Germany, but the killing continued informally as T-4 personnel were transferred to Nazi death camps such as Belzec, Sobibor, and Treblinka where they helped to build gas chambers. The full enormity of these crimes did not become public knowledge until 1946–1947, when twenty-three defendants (all but three of them physicians) were put on trial in Nuremberg in the so-called Doctors' Trial. To more than one historian, Aktion T-4 was the first Nazi mass-murder program to target specific groups of people, and thus was a "first chapter" to the "Final Solution"— the genocide of European Jews.[1]

This brutal chapter in German history warrants attention because not only has it tainted the word "euthanasia" ever since, it also shows that—the arguments of American euthanasia proponents notwithstanding—there were enough disturbing similarities between the two national versions of euthanasia to provide ESA critics with valuable propaganda. As later events would demonstrate, euthanasia opponents have sometimes used the *argumentum ad Hitlerum* irresponsibly, but some euthanasia supporters have been equally guilty of denying any comparisons between themselves and the Nazis.[2]

The origins of Nazi euthanasia, like those of the American euthanasia movement, predate the Third Reich and were intertwined with the history of eugenics and social Darwinism, and with efforts to discredit traditional morality and ethics. Nazi euthanasia "policies did not materialize out of thin air in response to unforeseeable wartime circumstances; they were entertained long in advance, by people who were very conscious of past precedents and of what they were doing."[3] Beginning in the late nineteenth century, German physicians and scientists increasingly used the language of eugenics and social Darwinism to characterize their approaches to public health. The result was "racial hygiene," roughly equivalent to what Anglo-Americans called eugenics. Racial hygiene was a form of preventive medicine that, by drawing heavily on Darwinist notions, attempted to balance the health needs of the individual and those of society.[4] Racial hygienists argued that such policies as health and disability insurance, the end of child labor, and the expansion of hospitals and clinics interfered with the process of natural selection that normally strengthened the species by eliminating its weaker members. Modern, civilized society needed a new science of public health that continued to protect the less fit with social security measures, while humanely doing the work of natural selection through eugenic programs designed to prevent the reproduction of inferior individuals.

By the beginning of the twentieth century, this Darwinian and eugenic viewpoint had gained an impressive list of converts.[5] Prominent German scientists cited the corrosive impact of Darwinism on ethics to justify challenging the traditional Christian prohibition against taking innocent human life. While some viewed euthanasia in terms of a right to die exercised by a mentally competent adult suffering from a terminal illness, this notion was often conflated with the belief in forcible killing of biologically deficient life. As happened during the debate over euthanasia in twentieth-century America, some turn-of-the-century Germans fudged the differences between voluntary and involuntary mercy killing for a host of reasons ranging from the humane to the economic and biological, without being terribly vexed by the philosophic distinctions between the two. Because the debate over euthanasia in early twentieth-century Germany and America invariably addressed its social dimensions, advocates for its legalization found it hard to resist arguing that terminally ill or disabled individuals should choose euthanasia in the interests of society, the human race, and their families. This theme of social justifications overshadowing individual choice extended beyond Germany and constituted a tension that characterized many arguments in favor of euthanasia in twentieth-century America.[6]

Before World War I, the most extensive debate over euthanasia fittingly took place in 1913 in the pages of Ernst Haeckel's *Das monistische Jahrhundert.* Some readers asked, What was the point of stoically suffering in the throes of a terminal illness when Haeckel's Monist League denied there was any afterlife? Why cannot a doctor put incurably ill patients out of their misery? Not everyone in the Monist League agreed that there was a right to a speedy, pain-free death, but there was little disagreement with the theory that all suffering diminished the individual by restricting his or her contribution to the community. In a day and age when scientific and medical discourse resonated with eugenic themes, it seemed as if every discussion of a right to die was fated to return to the question of what the dying person owed to society.[7]

World War I helped to transform euthanasia into a matter of compelling state interest in Germany. The carnage on the battlefield and the material deprivations of the home-front during and after the war compelled many Germans, especially in the medical profession, to turn their attention to national resources and the glaring contrast between a stoically suffering "healthy" nation and the thousands of handicapped individuals housed at state expense in special institutions. The severe provisions of the 1919 Versailles Peace Treaty exacerbated the national mood of anxiety over Germany's survival. When asylums refilled in the 1920s, the war continued to cast a sinister pall over German discussions about what to do with the nation's dependent citizens. Opinion makers emphasized the collective needs of the German people and their future generations, not the needs of individual patients.

A landmark tract, Alfred Hoche and Karl Binding's *Permitting the Destruction of Unworthy Life*, appeared in 1920 and brought the issue of euthanasia into sharper focus. Neither Binding, a professor of law, nor Hoche, a professor of psychiatry with a specialty in neuropathology, became Nazi ideologues, which made what they had to say about euthanasia all the more alarming. In effect, they provided the rationale for the later program of direct medical killing during the Third Reich.[8]

Karl Binding preferred to concentrate on the legal difficulties of putting euthanasia into practice. Starting from the position that every person had the freedom to commit suicide, he proceeded to justify voluntary euthanasia, then mercy killing of unconscious dying individuals, and finally the humane killing of state-dependent defectives. These latter were people whose lives were "not just absolutely worthless, but even of negative value."[9] They apparently had no will to either live or die and were terrible burdens on their families and society. They were "the fearsome counter image of true humanity . . . arous[ing] horror in nearly everyone who meets them." Their continued existence was a reproach to "the sacrifice of the finest flower of humanity" left strewn on the battlefields of World War I. According to Binding, they had forfeited the protection of the law, and their death, properly safeguarded, would be a godsend to everyone concerned. The benefits of legalized euthanasia would far outweigh the inevitable abuses.

Much like the American Humanist Charles Potter, Binding had begun by questioning "a sticking point in our moral and social outlook," moved to defending a consenting individual's right to die, and found himself at the end recommending the involuntary killing of incurable inmates of state hospitals. There was nothing inevitable in the progression of Binding's and Potter's thinking. But, equally, there is no evidence that either of them was brought kicking and screaming to this conclusion.[10]

Alfred Hoche, like Binding, urged a radical change in traditional morality and medical ethics. Convinced of the utter insignificance of individual experience in contrast to the power of biology and heredity, he was appalled at the expense of maintaining the roughly 30,000 "idiots" in German private and state institutions, at a yearly average cost of 1,300 marks per patient.[11] These people were "constitutionally less valuable elements" that could no longer be supported amid the grim conditions facing Germany after the war. To Hoche, the Hippocratic Oath, like conventional religious sentiments about the sanctity of life, had ceased to be relevant in post-1919 Germany, and he predicted that society would "eventually come to the conclusion that *eliminating those who are completely mentally dead is no crime, no immoral act, no emotional cruelty, but is rather a permissible and useful act.*" Like euthanasia advocates across the ocean heralding the overthrow of traditional ethics, Hoche was sure that history was on his side and that "a new age . . . operating with a higher morality" was dawning.[12]

Initially, Binding and Hoche failed to win many converts. In the years between the publication of their tract and the 1933 coming to power of the Nazis, critics of euthanasia tended to outnumber admirers. Physicians generally opposed euthanasia, citing the Hippocratic Oath or the risk to patients. But the advent of the Depression made it harder for psychiatrists specifically to resist calls for the enactment of euthanasia or eugenic laws. Between 1924 and 1929, the number of psychiatric patients in Weimar Germany rose from 185,397 to more than 300,000, and despite extensive efforts to release patients back into the community, the number of long-term, chronically ill patients jumped, turning most asylums into primarily custodial institutions. When cutbacks took effect after 1929, professional morale plummeted. Predictably, interest in eugenic sterilization swelled, although a majority of physicians still opposed it and euthanasia as late as the eve of the Nazi takeover.[13]

Adolf Hitler's rise to Germany's chancellorship in 1933 abruptly altered the country's cultural, social, and political climate. Overnight, eugenics and euthanasia virtually became approved state policies. In May 1933 the Nazis introduced a eugenic sterilization law that ultimately led to the asexualization of some 400,000 Germans, about 1 percent of the country's population. Following Hitler's own views, Germans were also encouraged to rid themselves of incurably sick "burdensome lives." In the 1930s, German filmmakers produced movies about the country's mentally and physically handicapped, the most notorious of which was the manipulative feature film titled *Ich klage an* (I accuse), released in 1941 with the approval of the Nazi state. Such films were intended to confuse the distinctions between patient self-determination and government-ordered, medicalized murder of the disabled.[14] All of a sudden Binding and Hoche's ideas were fashionable, and calls began for the "destruction of the mentally ill as lives unworthy of life." The growing impatience of Germans with the institutionalized mentally ill was mirrored in the remark of one young Schutzstaffeln (SS) visitor to the head psychiatrist of the Elfing-Haar asylum that the staff might as well place a machine gun at the hospital entrance and mow down the inmates.[15]

Apart from the convinced Nazis, most asylum physicians bent with the political winds and pledged allegiance to the new ideology of considering only "what serves the German nation." About half of all German physicians joined the Nazi Party and its adjunct organizations, including the SS. Psychiatrists had special reasons for entering a symbiotic relationship with the Nazi state. Despised as impotent to cure mental illness, psychiatrists found their interests lay in adopting pro-euthanasia rhetoric as the 1930s progressed and cooperating with the Nazis in enforcing the sterilization law. The result was that an estimated 30–40 percent of all Germans sterilized between 1934 and 1936 were asylum patients.[16]

Thus, by the time Hitler gave the go-ahead for the euthanasia campaign in 1939, the collective mentality of the country's psychiatrists and their institutional staff had been shaped to accept the killing of patients. In October 1939 Hitler issued a secret decree to start the killing, expanded by this point to include adults. Unlike the German sterilization law, the euthanasia edict was not strictly legal and was justified on the basis of the Führer's power over life and death in the Third Reich.[17]

The killing of sick and disabled children and adults within Germany started quickly, matched by the mass shootings of Jewish and Polish patients in the newly conquered regions of eastern Europe.

By early 1940 the first gassings of Polish and Jewish patients had taken place. Meanwhile, in German hospitals the selection of victims proceeded apace, and those diagnosed as "useless" were dispatched to the killing centers. Criteria for selection were supposed to be exact, but over time they were bent to include the old, infirm, and difficult, along with epileptics, schizophrenics, cripples, and the mentally retarded.

Just as Hitler's original order remained a secret, so the entire process was covert. False certificates of death were sent to victims' families, but eventually relatives and friends began to get suspicious. Patients alive one day were reported to have died weeks earlier. Some Germans clearly cared little about what happened to their institutionalized relatives, but many were appalled as the real state of affairs gradually became known. Protests ensued and the churches—especially the Roman Catholic clergy—began criticizing the government. Finally, in late August 1941 the Nazi leadership ordered the T-4 program terminated.

The official end to Aktion T-4 in 1941 simply meant that in German clinics and hospitals a sort of decentralized and unsystematic euthanasia unfolded, as patients were put to death by starvation, exhaustion from work, or lethal medicines. As T-4 personnel dispersed to the concentration and slave labor camps, the pace of murder actually accelerated. Criminals, orphans, the sick, the injured, and the racially undesirable were sent to the gas chambers. The killing did not stop until the end of the war. By then, this second stage of Nazi euthanasia had resulted in more deaths than the 70,000 to 90,000 accomplished in the first stage.

There was certainly nothing inevitable about the way early defenses of euthanasia culminated in the horrors of 1939–1945. Then, as now, it was perfectly possible for an individual to defend the voluntary right to die while opposing coercive euthanasia. The critical turning point in the German descent into medicalized brutality was the 1933 advent of the Nazi regime, more so than any spirited, pre–Third Reich endorsement of euthanasia. Nazification plunged the country into a social revolution and a world war that desensitized Germans in ways barely imaginable before 1933.[18] In extreme times, toleration of extreme measures is apt to rise, and some ordinary people will become extraordinary criminals.

However, Germans who expressed their support for euthanasia, no matter what their intentions, bear some responsibility for what followed, if only because they helped to acclimatize minds to the possibility of mercy killing. In that sense, there were striking similarities in the pro-euthanasia rhetoric on both sides of the Atlantic. Charles Potter, no less than Karl Binding or Alfred Hoche, was intent on ending what later activists would call the "conspiracy of silence" surrounding death and dying. Potter and other euthanasia backers were dedicated to dismantling the traditional moral and religious barriers to euthanasia, just as they had sought to dismantle the obstacles to eugenics and birth control. The Nazi euthanasia experience shows that lowering such barriers can be a risky business, if what replaces them provides no firm checks on baser human instincts. The conditions of total war from 1939 to 1945 made such risks exponentially worse.

As events after 1945 demonstrated, many Americans believed that legalizing active euthanasia started the country down a slippery slope. Within an altered cultural climate characterized by the dire warnings of religious leaders that moral errors were a threat to democracy, euthanasia proponents had only marginal success convincing Americans that mercy killing was not a lapse into Nazi barbarism but instead was a major victory in the battle for individual freedom.

II.

Although full disclosure of the Nazi euthanasia program awaited the end of the war, rumors of German atrocities against mental patients were confirmed in spring 1941.[19] The first reactions of euthanasia advocates are revealing. C. Killick Millard, secretary of the British VELS, believed incongruously that the reported fatalities taking place in Poland were actually "victims . . . driven to suicide."[20] When the reality became undeniable, the ESA's Ann Mitchell expressed unhappiness with Nazi methods but not with the results. Noting, in May 1940, that the Nazi doctors "gave the insane [Polish] children of several asylums morphine and then shot them," she added "[o]f course, this is a great blessing but it is too bad that it had to come about in just this way." In late 1941, she assured Millard that "[w]e all hate Hitler and know he must be defeated," but observed hopefully that the war would usher in a new "biological age," revolutionizing thinking so that mass sterilization and euthanasia would become acceptable. Publicly, however, Mitchell and the ESA issued a statement to the press in 1942 protesting the Nazi "wholesale slaughter of innocents." To prevent "any possible misunderstanding" of the ESA's agenda, the ESA reaffirmed its support for only voluntary euthanasia.[21]

By showing privately a fairly equivocal attitude toward Nazi euthanasia, Mitchell was not speaking for the whole ESA. Many members did indeed support only voluntary euthanasia. But there were elements in her thinking that are recognizable in the thought of other ESA stalwarts, such as Potter and Philbrick. All deplored Nazism, and once America entered the war they were solidly behind the Allied effort, recognizing Hitlerism as a danger to the democratic values they cherished. At the same time, their interpretations of euthanasia were not altogether unlike Nazi versions of euthanasia. One is led to wonder how Potter, Philbrick, and others would have reacted to Nazi euthanasia had German mercy killing started well before World War II, such as the Nazi sterilization program. Their official attitudes toward Nazi euthanasia were affected by the fact that their British colleagues in the VELS were at war with Hitler's Germany as early as September 1939, and sympathy toward Nazi euthanasia would have appeared insensitive. Then, after America's entry into the war in December 1941, there was the pressure to sound patriotic and condemn all policies of the Third Reich. Without that pressure, they might have shown considerably more enthusiasm for German euthanasia, as had American eugenicists after the 1933 Nazi sterilization law went into effect.[22]

Even as reports of Nazi barbarism were reaching the United States, the ESA struck a committee in 1943 that included Potter and feminist and birth control activist Jean Burnett Tompkins to draft a bill legalizing involuntary euthanasia for "idiots, imbeciles, and congenital monstrosities." Because the news from Europe grew grimmer, nothing came of the project. But it did indicate that most (if not all) early ESA members had few qualms about euthanasia for the nonconsenting handicapped.[23]

Charles Potter again stands out as someone who favored this form of euthanasia. For example, to justify the legalization of voluntary euthanasia he raised the prospect in 1943 of thousands of sick, wounded, and disabled soldiers returning home after the war, as they had after World War I. He predicted that many of them, "realizing that their own suffering is causing great anguish to their relatives and friends," would eventually beg society for a "merciful release" from their incurable injuries or interminable pain. By justifying euthanasia as a rational response to the horrible sacrifices made in both world wars, Potter sounded eerily like Binding and Hoche, as well as the Nazis who had viewed euthanasia as a practical solution to the severe overcrowding in state institutions. Of course, Potter assumed that this form of merciful death would be requested voluntarily by the veterans themselves; but his assumption that they would feel this way, once they realized the burden they were imposing on others, ran the decided risk of suggesting they had a duty to die.[24]

Sharing Potter's views on involuntary euthanasia was Eleanor Dwight Jones, ESA executive vice president from 1942 to her death in 1965 at the age of eighty-four. Jones was one of the biggest believers in the notion that the legalization of euthanasia constituted the next great liberation for Americans in the wake of women's suffrage, the 1936 *One Package* court ruling on birth control, and the enactment of eugenic sterilization laws. Jones, another Unitarian, was a dedicated, indefatigable worker for whatever cause she espoused. She occupied a mainly self-effacing role at the ESA, for many years doing most of its clerical work and rejecting all offers to serve as president. In its early years, the ESA had a tiny budget and few members able to volunteer their services, so Jones *was* the ESA and deserves as much credit as Potter for what she did for the euthanasia movement.[25]

Jones's involvement in the eugenics and birth control movements dated back to the interwar period. President of the American Birth Control League (ABCL) between 1928 and 1935, Jones left many birth control activists believing that her feuds with Margaret Sanger had hindered the progress of the movement to decriminalize contraception. Described as a "martinet," and more politely as belonging to "that group of Angry Young Women which is said to begin with Harriet Beecher Stowe and end with Mary McCarthy," Jones was a fervent admirer of Potter, praising the Humanist Society he founded and periodically appearing publicly with him during the 1930s. Her migration from the women's suffrage campaign to the eugenics and birth control movements, and then to the ESA, was a signature career pattern for many American women social reformers between the 1920s and 1960s, underlining the philosophic connections among all four movements.

In the 1940s Jones and Margaret Sanger, despite their personal disagreements, found a common home in the ESA. Jones liked nothing better than to quote Sanger, who once said that the euthanasia and birth control movements were highly similar, "one being to bring entrance into life under control of reason, and the other to bring the exit of life under that control."[26] But no matter how strong her interest in eugenics and birth control, Jones experienced her greatest satisfaction working for legalized euthanasia.[27] At the same time, she knew that the war years were the wrong time to press for such reforms, and so the ESA suspended all legislative activity in 1943. Once the war ended, however, Jones threw herself into mobilizing legislative support for voluntary euthanasia in the hopes that it would serve as a springboard for a later involuntary euthanasia bill, and she targeted New York State as the first site for such an endeavor.

Jones's aim was to secure a bill legalizing elective euthanasia by presenting petitions—signed by clergymen and physicians—to the New York State legislature. She worked closely with gynecologist Robert Latou Dickinson, ESA president from 1946 until his death in 1950. Dickinson, born in 1861 in Brooklyn, New York, was a pioneering champion of sex education, marriage counseling, and the use of rubber and plastic pelvic models for medical teaching purposes.[28] Dickinson also played a critical role in the birth control movement, working tirelessly to get the medical profession to recognize the health benefits of contraception. Although he (like Jones) had a troubled relationship with Sanger, he shared the latter's opinions about the value of sex education and the emancipating potential of informed and accessible family planning.[29]

Dickinson and Jones largely typified the ESA in the 1940s. Whether it was euthanasia, birth control, marriage counseling, or sex education, Dickinson, like Jones, saw them all as means for liberating human beings from the ravages of illness, disability, aging, and ignorance about the physiology of sex and reproduction. Dickinson's personal goal, as he put it, was simply to improve the individual's quality of life. Medically supervised euthanasia was another weapon in the struggle to enhance the quality of life and end human suffering.[30]

Following a pattern set by early ESA members, Dickinson's interest in birth control spilled over into eugenics. In 1943 he joined Birthright, a eugenic organization in everything but name, founded by the social worker Marian Olden.[31] Olden had helped to found Birthright in 1937 and had lobbied unsuccessfully for a state sterilization

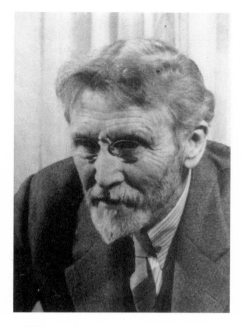

Robert Latou Dickinson. *Francis A. Countway Library of Medicine, Boston.*

law in New Jersey.[32] Dickinson was the first chairman of Birthright's Medical and Scientific Committee, originally formed in 1949, and in 1950, Birthright's national office was switched from Princeton to Dickinson's studio at the New York Academy of Medicine. His involvement in Birthright was just another example of the close affinity between the euthanasia and eugenic movements in America and elsewhere, and the common effort to break down physicians' official resistance to euthanasia and sterilization as standard medical techniques. Because physicians illicitly performed both practices, Dickinson reasoned, there was no reason not to publicly endorse them.[33]

Dickinson's interest in euthanasia was less consuming than Jones's, but he still defended it with his customary zest. With Jones, he looked beyond simply legalizing voluntary euthanasia to a time when, he hoped, society would contemplate merciful, involuntary euthanasia for incurable defectives, rather than waste tax-payer-supported social services on them. This would free up resources that might instead be "allotted to children or adults who could be of value to the community," he told a CBS radio audience in 1946. To those who questioned why the state should hold such power of life or death over its citizens, Dickinson answered that the state already "selects its healthiest citizens to expose to slaughter and life-long maiming to release others from greater ills. Why deny it the power to end life that is not worth living?"[34]

Dickinson's main contribution to the euthanasia movement was his chairmanship in the late 1940s of the ESA-affiliated "Committee of 1776 Physicians for Legalization of Voluntary Euthanasia in New York State." The committee produced a petition signed by 1,776 New York State physicians, urging each state legislator to introduce an elective euthanasia bill for anyone incurably ill and over twenty-one years of age who wished a doctor to end his or her life painlessly. By late 1947 every member of the state legislature had received a copy.[35]

The so-called Committee of 1776, so impressive on paper, turned into a public relations nightmare for the ESA. Next to winning the approval of America's religious leaders, the ESA's board most wanted to win the endorsement of the country's medical profession. But medical organizations across the country implored state politicians to ignore the petition, condemning the idea of legalized mercy killing.[36] In 1950, the American Medical Association (AMA) issued a statement that the "majority of doctors do not believe in [euthanasia]."[37] State and national medical societies' denunciations of euthanasia packed considerable punch since membership in such organizations and the AMA held the key to hospital privileges and patient referrals as well as malpractice liability protection. Physicians who defied the professional orthodoxy on euthanasia stood to be penalized heavily. Even President Franklin D. Roosevelt admitted that "[w]e can't go up against the State Medical Societies; we just can't do it."[38]

Predictably, some of the doctors whose names appeared on the petition complained to the ESA that they had never signed in the first place, or had misunderstood the meaning of the petition, or had signed and had then undergone a change of heart. In some cases this was due to a backlash from their patients. In other cases it was due to threats that they would lose ward privileges at—and have to sever their connections to—Catholic hospitals, tactics used by these hospitals to intimidate physicians associated with the ESA or birth control organizations and clinics.[39] As one signatory complained in 1948, his medical practice had "fallen off 1,000 dollars per month" since his name was leaked to the press.[40]

These factors later helped to hinder similar efforts in New Jersey to enlist physicians' support for euthanasia. There, an ESA-backed petition signed by 166 doctors eventually made its way to the state legislature in 1957. However, the campaign ground to a halt when the Archdiocese of Newark published the names of all state signatories. The Medical Society of New Jersey joined the attack, stating that "the practice of euthanasia has been and continues to be in conflict with accepted principles of morality and sound medical practice."[41]

Undoubtedly, some of the physicians who protested the public release of their names had signed the Committee of 1776 petition hurriedly without either reading or thinking about it carefully. Others just as obviously knew what they were doing but had not anticipated the kind of trouble they would incur. Some doctors demanded that their names be withdrawn from the list and resigned their committee memberships. As one physician testily told Dickinson in 1948, "[t]he recent release which your publicity agent gave to the press including my own name and others in the community has caused us unlimited amount of embarrassment. I do not care to have anything to do with this movement."[42]

Even when physicians were sympathetic toward some forms of euthanasia, their cultural status and self-perception in the postwar years made it awkward for them to support mercy killing. Doing so conveyed the impression that physicians were unable to cure illness, a distinctly unflattering image at a time when confidence in medical science's ability to find cures for disease—especially cancer—was growing steadily. Indeed, the histories of the euthanasia movement and the national crusade to find a cure for cancer in the twentieth century were intimately intertwined. Stories about slow, painful deaths from cancer were often cited by proponents of euthanasia as reasons for choosing suicide, as was the increasing number of people who developed cancer.[43]

However, these stories did not sit well with many physicians. William S. McCann, a University of Rochester (New York) professor of medicine and member of the ESA, accused the group of fear mongering about the pain associated with a cancer patient's death. Contending that with the use of surgery and analgesic drugs he could control a cancer patient's pain, McCann asserted in 1952 that the "vast majority of cancer deaths are painless. Death from cancer is, generally speaking, no more unpleasant that most other forms of death, and I object to the many public agencies that persist in singling out cancer and building up so much fear of it that people are made ill thereby."[44] McCann's reaction to ESA literature illustrates the ambivalent nature of physicians' opinions about euthanasia. While they saw a need in certain cases for ending dying patients' lives when they became too painful, they were extremely leery about the professional implications of officially endorsing such practices.

McCann's views were largely consistent with popular and official attitudes toward cancer. What had been viewed in the interwar period with dread, loathing, and an almost paralyzing fear, after World War II was thought of increasingly with hope that scientists would discover a cure for cancer. Led by the National Cancer Institute and the American Cancer Society, Americans began expecting better health and looking to their doctors for the goods and services necessary for an improved quality of life.

The inevitable disillusionment stemming from these high expectations of the medical profession materialized in the 1960s. Until then, however, physicians enjoyed an enviable status, one that conflicted with the image of doctors helping patients to die. TV characters such as Ben Casey and Dr. Kildare reflected public confidence in the power of medicine. Privately, doctors often withheld treatment from dying patients or eased them out of their misery. Publicly, however, they tended to dodge the issue and stand behind their profession's position that the doctor's goal was to try to keep patients alive, not hasten their departure from this world. In a cultural climate stressing an imminent cure for cancer, and doctors doing more rather than less for their patients, the ESA's petition in favor of euthanasia simply did not resonate with a lot of Americans, physicians and patients alike.[45]

ESA-orchestrated petitions supporting euthanasia attracted even more bad press when well-publicized mercy killings hit the headlines in the late 1940s. For example, on 30 September 1949 Carol Paight, a twenty-year-old Connecticut college student, shot her fifty-two-year-old father while he lay unconscious in a hospital bed after exploratory surgery. Paight, allegedly in a kind of fugue mental state, had used her father's police revolver after she learned that he was incurably ill with cancer. He never gained consciousness after the shooting and took about seven hours to die. Though her defense rested on the insanity plea, she was reported to have said just before the shooting that she had to do something to keep her father from knowing that he had only six painful weeks to live. Paight, an attractive young woman, whom cameras frequently caught sobbing softly over her father's fate, went on trial and was acquitted on 8 February 1950. She cut a highly sympathetic figure, something euthanasia advocates exploited in their official comments on the case.

An even more publicized euthanasia case was that of Dr. Hermann Sander, a family physician from the town of Candia, near Manchester, New Hampshire. Sander became the first physician in American history to stand trial for mercy killing, charged with administering lethal injections to a woman dying of cancer on the morning of 4 December 1949. Sander, a beloved doctor renowned for his selflessness and generosity, never denied that he had injected air intravenously into his patient's arm. The patient, a fifty-nine-year-old housewife whose weight had dropped from 140 to 80 pounds, could no longer eat and had developed resistance to the large doses of painkillers the hospital staff had given her to ease her suffering.

Sander's trial opened on 20 February 1950 and quickly became a media circus. Covered by more than 100 reporters from around the United States and the world, it generated almost as much commentary as the 1935 trial of Bruno Richard Hauptmann for the kidnap-murder of the Lindbergh baby and reminded Americans of yet another famous court trial: *Time* magazine, noting the size of the press corps that descended on southern New Hampshire, asked, "Not Since Scopes?"[46] Dozens and dozens of editorials weighed the pros and cons of Sander's actions. He was condemned by evangelist Billy Graham and Richard J. Cushing, the Roman Catholic Archbishop of Boston. But Sander also had his backers, including Earnest Hooten, the Harvard anthropologist and eugenicist. Dorothy Kenyon, a lawyer, ESA advisory council member, American Civil Liberties Union board member, birth control activist, and former delegate to the United Nations Commission on the Status of Women, also rallied to Sander's side, as did C. Killick Millard, the VELS, and a group of twenty-two Unitarian ministers. Charles Potter called Sander a "martyr," and Eleanor Dwight Jones declared the Sander case proof that New Hampshire had to legalize euthanasia.[47]

Despite the fact that the Manchester area had a sizable Catholic population, an all-male jury, satisfied that the patient was dead at the time of the lethal injection, acquitted Sander on 10 March 1950. Sander's own relief with the verdict was greatly tempered when on 19 April 1950 the State Board of Registration in Medicine unanimously voted to revoke his license to practice.[48] The State Board restored his license two months later, but in the meantime Sander, out of work and heavily in debt, had to perform manual labor for neighbors. He had to wait until December 1954 before he was granted his old hospital privileges.

The Sander and Paight trials presented the ESA with opportunities to drum up support for its cause. In November 1949 Eleanor Dwight Jones and Charles Potter hurried to Stamford, Connecticut, and with local help were able to establish an ESA state chapter on 8 January 1950, called the Voluntary Euthanasia Society of Connecticut (VESC). Evidence of the strong links between the birth control and euthanasia movements resurfaced in the formation of the Connecticut chapter. Connecticut had long been a battleground for activists seeking the repeal of state laws prohibiting contraception. Its 1879 statute, masterminded by Phineas T. Barnum, the circus promoter and temperance militant, had outlawed both the sale and use of birth control devices. Not until 1965 was the law finally overturned by the U.S. Supreme Court in its pioneering *Griswold v. Connecticut* ruling, thanks in large part to the persistent efforts of Connecticut birth control activists. Some of the individuals instrumental in that struggle joined the VESC, including Julie Howson, Harriet Janney, and Hilda Crosby Standish.[49]

In 1959 the VESC managed to get a voluntary euthanasia bill, patterned closely after the New York State model law, introduced in the state legislature. The bill, authorizing euthanasia for anyone over twenty-one years of age and of sound mind who was suffering from a disease medical science could not cure, left unclear whether a physician had to administer the lethal dose. It was similarly ambiguous about whether individuals suffering from conditions such as multiple sclerosis or polio could petition for euthanasia. For these and other reasons it went down to a decisive defeat.[50]

In the meantime, the ESA had been even less lucky in New Hampshire. Jones traveled to Manchester and attempted to found a New Hampshire chapter of the ESA. While she managed to enlist the support of several distinguished local individuals, state opinion was far too polarized over the Sander case. A volunteer worker told Jones that the situation in New Hampshire was "so fouled up that the time is not ripe to push legalized euthanasia." ESA representatives were also disappointed that Sander refused to speak out in favor of euthanasia. By late 1950 any momentum gathered from the Sander trial had petered out in New Hampshire, and ESA hopes of forming a state chapter had evaporated.[51]

The fallout from the Sander and Paight trials taught euthanasia advocates another tough lesson. They learned they had to be extremely careful about what they said regarding well-publicized mercy killings. On the one hand, the ESA welcomed the press coverage of the Paight and Sander trials because it personalized the euthanasia issue, describing the experiences of real human beings suffering under all-too-familiar circumstances and having to make enormously difficult decisions in the face of ages-old value systems. At the very least, the trials prompted discussion of euthanasia, both pro and con, proving that even bad publicity was better than none at all.[52]

On the other hand, there was a decided risk that defending Sander and Paight meant endorsing the mercy killing of people whose desire to die was questionable at best. As critics noted, Paight's father had never asked his daughter to shoot him, and the fact that he took so long to die hardly betokened a speedy and humane death. Nor had Sander's patient ever asked him to kill her.[53] Indeed, the news of Sander's arrest had compelled Dickinson and the Committee of 1776 to issue a denial that they stood for anything but voluntary euthanasia, nor did they encourage breaking the law. The committee's goal was the "amendment" of the laws to permit safeguarded voluntary euthanasia for incurable patients, not their violation. However, that too merely raised the question of what the actions of Hermann Sander and Carol Paight had to do with the goals of the euthanasia movement. If the ESA and its English counterpart the VELS defended only a "right to die," not a "right to kill," why then did they not denounce what Sander and Paight had done? Until euthanasia proponents could answer these questions, there was little chance of attracting large numbers of Americans to the cause. Americans might empathize with what Paight and Sander had done, but they were reluctant to see it legalized.[54]

III.

The imbroglio over the Committee of 1776 confirmed again that much of the opposition facing the ESA came from the medical profession. However, no American groups did more to contest the legalization of euthanasia than the country's organized churches in general and the Roman Catholic Church in particular. Indeed, by the end of the 1940s euthanasia advocates were engaged in nothing less than a culture war with the American Catholic hierarchy and most mainstream Protestant churches, a conflict that stretched far beyond the euthanasia issue itself to encompass issues such as governmental aid to parochial schools, the "wall of separation" between church and state, and the very nature of democratic citizenship. This conflict between the Catholic Church and defenders of euthanasia was nothing new; it had surfaced during the Bollinger baby episode and in the 1930s. But its intensity in the late 1940s was unprecedented, if only because each side in the battle believed nothing less than the future of America was at stake.

The intensity of this struggle was heightened considerably by the fact that it occurred against the backdrop of the developing Cold War between the United States and the Soviet Union. As anticommunist sentiments rose in the late 1940s and peaked in the early 1950s during the McCarthy era, American liberals who sympathized with the euthanasia cause watched with dismay as their religious opponents conflated support for communism with enthusiasm for euthanasia. Already reeling from accusations that the ESA favored Nazi-like measures, the organization struggled valiantly but in vain to defend itself in the 1950s.

The euthanasia movement's campaign to win over American public opinion would have been considerably easier had it not coincided with a period in U.S. history that saw the Roman Catholic Church become "the dominant cultural institution in the country."[55] From the 1930s to the mid-1950s, the Church enjoyed a unity, rigor, power, and influence that propelled it to the very center of American life. What made its cultural, political, and social muscle all the more impressive was the fact that only a generation earlier the Church had been viewed with deep-seated distrust by many Protestant Americans, a legacy of religious conflict that dated as far back as the sixteenth-century Reformation. Anti-Catholicism was also due to the fierce xenophobia of nativist Americans toward immigrants from Ireland and Italy who arrived in waves between the 1830s and 1920s. These anti-Catholic feelings helped defeat the Catholic Democratic Party candidate Al Smith in the presidential election of 1928.

Widespread anti-Catholicism seemed to evaporate in the 1930s and 1940s; it was replaced by a diffuse public willingness to follow the Church's lead in setting the policy agenda for the country. This was partly due to the expansion in Catholicism's share of the nation's population, which, between 1930 and 1960, grew from 19 to 23 percent. Most Catholics lived in large urban areas, such as New York, Philadelphia, Chicago, and Boston. Brooklyn itself held more than one million Catholics in 1930.[56] Urban politicians, intimidated by the ballot-box might of Catholic voters, courted powerful Catholic prelates such as Francis Cardinal Spellman, whose chancery in New York was nicknamed "the powerhouse," and Cardinal Dennis Dougherty, who had the honor of offering the invocation at both the Republican and Democratic presidential nominating conventions in 1948. In states such as Connecticut the Catholic grip on politics was especially tight.[57]

Everything from movies to television reflected the formidable presence of the Church in daily life. Catholics monitored Hollywood films for over two decades, pressuring the studios to eliminate scenes of sex and violence from their movies. On television, Bishop Fulton J. Sheen's *Life Is Worth Living* show in the mid-1950s attracted an audience that outstripped even that of comedian Milton Berle's *Texaco Comedy Hour.* Little wonder that the Protestant *Christian Century* ran an eight-part series in 1944–1945, opening with the question: "Can Catholicism Win America?"[58]

American secular liberals worried about Catholicism's mainstream status in the 1940s because they remembered all too well the Church's steady support for Francisco Franco's right-wing nationalists in the Spanish Civil War, an event that many liberals and leftists saw as a dress rehearsal for World War II. They also remembered the speeches of the "radio priest" Charles Coughlin during the Depression, and how they became increasingly anti-Semitic and pro-Nazi after Coughlin's break with President Franklin D. Roosevelt in 1936.[59] Even anticommunist liberals were suspicious when, in the early 1950s, so many American Catholics applauded the efforts of Senator Joseph McCarthy to root out communists from government and other public institutions. Despite the effusive patriotism of American Catholics when the United States entered World War II in 1941, many liberals were convinced that the politics of the Catholic Church were a perennial threat to the personal freedoms they identified with American democracy.[60]

No issue seemed to represent the pernicious influence of Catholicism over individual freedom more than the teaching of the Church on sex. In 1930 Pope Pius XI issued the Vatican's first modern statement on sex and birth control, describing contraception as "an offense against the law of God and of nature" and those who practiced birth control as grave sinners. According to the Church, abstinence from the sex act was the only approved method of birth control; by nature conjugal acts were for begetting children above all else. Sex for pleasure was tantamount to masturbation. However, many Americans—Catholic and non-Catholic alike—were coming to a very different conclusion. They were growing convinced of the need to separate sex from reproduction and to plan the number of children they wished to raise.[61]

Church teaching on sex may have looked positively medieval to anti-Catholic liberals, but in fact it was in flux during the middle third of the twentieth century against a background of striking developments in science. Studies in the 1920s had demonstrated the existence of fertile and infertile periods each month in the female menstrual cycle. Then, in the 1940s, Alfred Kinsey published his findings on human sexual behavior, allegedly documenting high rates of homosexuality as well as premarital and extramarital sex for women and men.[62] By the 1950s the view started to take shape in American popular culture that denying one's sexual urges led to emotional or nervous disorders and that the judicious use of prophylactics could improve marital relations.[63] For Catholics, this trend was highlighted in 1951 when Pius XII approved of marriage partners planning their sex acts around the wife's cycle, the so-called rhythm method. However, Pope Paul VI's *Humanae Vitae* (1968) dashed the hopes of reformers and merely confirmed to the Church's detractors that modern medicine and science had rendered its ethical teachings on sex and reproduction seriously out-of-date. It was easy for those who castigated Vatican policy on sex to equate Catholic opposition to euthanasia with the church's seemingly irrational stand on birth control, which helps to account for the disproportionate numbers of birth control advocates within the euthanasia movement.[64]

Making matters worse for critics of the Church was the fact that American Catholicism's heyday coincided with the country's robust religiosity of the 1950s. Congress deferred to this revival of religious sentiment by adding the words "under God" to the Pledge of Allegiance and the phrase "in God we trust" to all United States currency. President Dwight D. Eisenhower regularly opened cabinet meetings with a prayer. Evangelical and fundamentalist churches enjoyed a remarkable growth after World War II, proof that the 1925 Scopes trial had not triggered a decline in fundamentalist Christianity. Evangelist Billy Graham and the Reverend Norman Vincent Peale, along with Bishop Sheen, spoke to receptive audiences numbering in the millions over radio and in newspapers and books. This "new piety" struck some observers as bland and theologically challenged, but there was no discounting how, as a new "civic religion" suspicious of radical ideas, it reversed whatever broad social, political, or cultural trends had been working in the euthanasia movement's favor since the Depression.[65]

Thus, nothing could have been more poorly timed than the ESA-sponsored 1948 statement (with Dickinson as its "ringleader") declaring euthanasia perfectly ethical, signed by fifty religious leaders from New York State.[66] Since its inception, the ESA had found it exceedingly difficult to recruit support from Protestant and Jewish clergymen who, like physicians, either objected strenuously in principle to euthanasia or feared repercussions if they demonstrated any sympathy toward it. Consequently, the statement on the ethical nature of euthanasia, later signed by a total of 379 Protestant and Jewish clergymen, represented a genuine breakthrough for the ESA, for it argued that there were no sound religious or moral reasons to prevent New York State from legalizing voluntary euthanasia. The clergymen's statement declared that elective euthanasia, "under the proper safeguards," was "medically indicated" and also "in accord with the most civilized and humane ethics and the highest concepts and practices of religion." Based on their experiences tending to the sick and dying, the clergymen rehearsed the arguments favored by many Unitarians and Humanists that painful and protracted death had no redeeming features and led only to "the degradation and disintegration of personality." The "sacredness of the human personality" required that individuals be granted a "right to die." As the clergymen concluded, by granting this right, society was simply "showing the same mercy to human beings as to the sub-human animal kingdom."[67]

Unsurprisingly, fully twenty out of the fifty clergymen who signed the New York petition were pastors at Unitarian/Universalist churches. Others among the fifty belonged to the liberal Union Theological Seminary of New York City, individuals such as W. Russell

Bowie, Henry Sloan Coffin, David E. Roberts, and Henry P. Van Dusen. Guy Emery Shipler, editor of *The Churchman*, a liberal monthly magazine unofficially aligned with the Episcopal Church, was also a signatory. As was the case with other euthanasia proponents, these clergymen were drawn to the movement for diverse reasons. But one common denominator was the belief that, in opposing the right to die, Roman Catholicism posed a distinct threat to American democracy.

If one individual stood out among the pro-euthanasia ministers it was Harry Emerson Fosdick, author of the popular *Christianity and Progress* (1922). Fosdick came to national prominence in the mid-1920s as a strident opponent of fundamentalist Christianity and, by the Depression, was, "by far, the best-known liberal [Protestant] minister in America, even in a sense a celebrity."[68]

Fosdick's allegiances to euthanasia, eugenics, and birth control typified an entire generation of euthanasia advocates, born in the waning years of the nineteenth century. Fosdick embraced the theory of evolution as an undergraduate at Colgate; he decided that his life's work lay in reconciling Christianity and the march of science. In full retreat from orthodoxy and rebelling against biblical literalism, he went on to study at the freethinking Union Theological Seminary, which, he wrote later, "offered a kind of intellectual liberty in the study of religion of which I had dreamed." Union Theological Seminary helped to turn Fosdick into a tireless supporter of the social gospel, the conviction that Christians had to do something about the unjust social conditions that "impinge on personality with frightful consequences." For Fosdick, one such unjust social condition was the prohibition against euthanasia.[69]

In 1925 Fosdick accepted John D. Rockefeller Jr.'s invitation to become head pastor of what ultimately became the Riverside Church, located next to Union Theological Seminary and Columbia University, and later home to pro-euthanasia Unitarian ministers John H. Lathrop and Donald McKinney. Fosdick retired from the pulpit in 1946 but remained a force in public life for many years, writing, lecturing, appearing on radio, and hobnobbing with presidents and statesmen.[70]

Fosdick's approach to religion, like Charles Potter's, was tinged with a curious mix of liberalism and paternalism. Fosdick insisted that Christianity be "intellectually hospitable, open-minded, liberty-loving, fair, [and] tolerant" and made sure that the Riverside Church was open to everyone, regardless of creed or formal confession. He combined these convictions with equally firm opinions about eugenics, euthanasia, and population control. An early member of the ESA, Fosdick had been one of the first ministers in America to publicly declare that voluntary euthanasia was not contrary to the principles of Christianity.[71] At the same time, Fosdick was a member of Marian Olden's Birthright, Inc., sharing her theory that "scientific eugenics" and "selective sterilization" of the mentally retarded were crucial to solving the problem of global overpopulation. In his opinion, eugenics, euthanasia, birth control, and population control were the kinds of causes that a humane, tolerant, scientifically informed, and public-spirited Christian ought to support.[72]

Fosdick's religious allies in the ESA included Henry Sloane Coffin, Guy Emery Shipler, and John Howland Lathrop. During the early stages of the Cold War, this group crusaded for the legalization of euthanasia, but their advocacy was interwoven with the larger campaign of American liberals to contest the power of the Catholic Church in public life. To them, support for euthanasia was not simply a just cause in itself; it was also a meaningful expression of the movement to create the self-determining personality type necessary to defend American democracy in the face of growing totalitarian challenges. Defending the individual's right to die was synonymous with scientific enlightenment and responsible democratic citizenship in an age many American intellectuals claimed was gripped by a crisis over personal freedom. Coffin, Fosdick, Shipler, and Lathrop agreed with Eleanor Dwight Jones, who asserted that the legalization of voluntary euthanasia was an affirmation of the "separation of church and state." "The [euthanasia] law we propose," she announced in 1949, "would leave each religious group free to follow the teachings of its own religion—in fact is merely in accord with the American ideal of religious freedom." Through its opposition to worthwhile measures such as euthanasia and birth control, the Catholic Church violated "the American ideal of religious freedom" by engaging in an "effort to dominate the rest of us," she warned in 1948. Hailing the formation that year of Protestants and Other Americans United for the Separation of Church and State (POAU), Jones declared the time had come to defeat Catholic political power.[73]

To ESA vice president Coffin, endorsing euthanasia was a similarly logical decision given his firm opinions about the Catholic Church and his staunch opposition to Christian fundamentalism. A one-time moderator of the Presbyterian Church, Coffin was also president emeritus of Union Theological Seminary and a self-styled liberal modernist. After studying at Union Theological Seminary and being ordained as a Presbyterian minister in 1900, he gained notoriety in 1925 for defending Fosdick's right to preach as an independent at First Presbyterian Church in New York City. He viewed the right to die as a fundamental liberty that all citizens in a genuine democracy should enjoy. The Catholic Church's refusal to legalize this right, Coffin insisted, was a denial of individual Catholics' freedom to think and do as they wished as well as an assault on the principle of separation of church and state. He was so alarmed about Catholicism that, in 1949, he claimed distinguishing between "totalitarian Moscow" and "totalitarian Rome" was virtually impossible. "If the one makes us tremble for American liberties, what of the other?" he asked.[74]

Guy Emery Shipler, an Episcopal minister, responded readily when in 1947 Eleanor Dwight Jones invited him and Coffin to become ESA vice presidents. "Our great need today," Jones stated, "is for strong Protestant cooperation to counter-balance the Catholic opposition."[75] Shipler agreed, and through his editorship of the militantly anti-Catholic *The Churchman* he attacked "the political encroachments of the Roman Catholic hierarchy" and lavished warm praise on POAU. Having signed the petition of 379 Protestant and Jewish ministers of New York State in favor of voluntary euthanasia, Shipler made sure that euthanasia received good reviews in the pages of *The Churchman*. How wedded Shipler was to purely elective euthanasia was never clear, given that in 1940 his magazine had published Earnest A. Hooten's disturbing defense of euthanasia as both a voluntary and involuntary eugenic measure.[76]

As the ESA's campaign to enlist the backing of American clergymen peaked, Paul Blanshard's 1949 best-seller *American Freedom and Catholic Power* was published. Blanshard was yet another recruit to the euthanasia cause who lumped it with eugenics, birth control, sex education, and nonsectarian schooling as issues whose vigorous defense was equivalent to defending democracy itself. Blanshard was a trustee of the Ethical Culture Society and one-time Congregationalist minister who did graduate studies at the Union Theological Seminary. He served as an urban reformer in the La Guardia administration in New York City in the 1930s, and during World War

II he was an economic analyst and consultant at the State Department.

Blanshard's *American Freedom and Catholic Power* contained blistering attacks on the "anti-democratic," "intolerant," "totalitarian," and positively "un-American" nature of Catholicism. Blanshard condemned the Catholic Church for frustrating Birthright's attempts to persuade state legislators to enact eugenic sterilization laws. "Meanwhile," Blanshard wrote, "the feeble-minded who are at large in our population produce future Americans at a much faster rate than our normal citizens."[77] He also attacked the Catholic leadership for opposing the ESA's legislative efforts, at the same time lauding the ESA's "humane" support for the safeguarded right of Americans to seek a "merciful release." To Blanshard, the controversy over euthanasia was a typical example of uninformed, authoritarian Catholic interference in the private lives of democratic citizens. Naturally, the ESA hailed his book as "a brilliant and scholarly study of the menacing encroachment of the Roman Catholic Church in the fields of education, medicine, and sex morals."[78]

Blanshard proved to be the linchpin of the anti-Catholic coalition in favor of euthanasia, holding together its religious and secular wings. Perhaps the best known of the secular liberals was Horace Kallen, an ESA advisory council member and one of the cofounders of the New School for Social Research. Kallen, born in Germany in 1882, was the son of a Hebrew scholar and Orthodox rabbi. In 1905 he was dismissed from his teaching post at Princeton for being an avowed unbeliever, and in 1918 the University of Wisconsin fired him for being a pacifist. These setbacks reinforced his passionate belief in intellectual liberty and freedom of speech. A philosopher, Kallen authored more than thirty books and countless articles and pamphlets, defending humanist ideas and the pluralist concept that each ethnic group has a unique contribution to make to American culture. He looked toward an interventionist state and its heavy reliance on public administration and secular education to eradicate the "religious establishments and political orders" that he thought undermined "government by the people."[79]

In 1956 Kallen, borrowing freely from Humanist philosophy, argued that what separated human beings from animals was precisely the ability to recognize that an individual whose consciousness was compromised by intense pain was better off dead than alive. "The principle and practice of euthanasia," he wrote, "seem to me among the consummations of the humanity of man, the ultimate step of his differentiation from the organic animalhood in which it roots." Kallen contended that one's very humanity rested on the recognition of this notion, suggesting that sufferers of incurable disease ought to choose euthanasia or have it chosen for them.[80]

Kallen's interest in euthanasia ultimately was inseparable from his fear of the threat he imagined the Roman Catholic Church posed for American democracy. In 1957, claiming he had been an ESA member "from the beginning," he lauded it for being "committed to a cause which every human being who has a spark of feeling should share," and for "struggling against [the] characteristically blind and fearful forces of reaction," what he called "the Romanist opposition." In 1958 he was the principal speaker at the ESA's twentieth anniversary annual meeting. To Kallen, euthanasia was first and foremost a "human rights" issue.[81]

His views were akin to those of Freda Kirchwey (1893–1976), editor of *The Nation* and a member of the ESA advisory council. Under her editorship, *The Nation* ran several pro-euthanasia stories and, in 1948, published portions of Blanshard's book under the title *The Roman Catholic Church in Medicine, Sex, and Education*. The efforts of organized religion—Catholic or otherwise—to deny Americans the right to die looked to liberals such as Kallen and Kirchwey like violations of the constitutional no-man's-land, which they imagined stretched between secular and religious society. If one believed in a pluralist democracy based on the concept of an inalienable personal right to define one's own existence, then defending the freedom to determine the conditions of one's own death was the obligation of every tolerant citizen.[82]

More radically liberal than Kallen and Kirchwey was the journal *The Truth Seeker*. Begun as a tabloid newspaper in 1873, *The Truth Seeker* was (by its own account) a "militantly atheist" publication that Robert Ingersoll, Clarence Darrow, H. L. Mencken, and Margaret Sanger had either written for or supported. Like Humanism and Ethical Culture, *The Truth Seeker* was devoted to "science," "free thought," and "whatever tends to elevate and emancipate the human race," and opposed "ecclesiasticism, dogmas, creeds, . . . and everything that degrades or burdens mankind mentally or physically." Not surprisingly, it took a strong pro-euthanasia position. "Science should wipe out life when life offers nothing but prolonged agony," it stated in 1949.[83]

The anti-Catholicism of ESA members Kallen, Coffin, Jones, Blanshard, and Shipler, and publications such as *The Truth Seeker*, was based on a deep distrust of the church's hierarchy, its congregation, and its teaching. Although individuals such as Blanshard always claimed they were attacking church leadership rather than lay Catholics and thus were free of antireligious bigotry, the fact that they saved their animosity for Catholicism rather than the medical profession, an equally stalwart opponent of euthanasia, signaled an inability to liberate themselves entirely from long-standing American anti-Catholic sentiment.

Their anti-Catholicism, however, did not occur in a vacuum. Whatever visceral prejudices these individuals harbored only partially explain the tenor of their comments about the Church's place in American society. Much of their anti-Catholicism was a reaction to the virulent attacks Catholic spokespersons launched in the 1940s and 1950s against supporters of euthanasia, birth control, eugenics, and population control. Anti-Catholicism was a backlash against the refusal of Church prelates such as Francis Cardinal Spellman of New York to recognize a strict separation of church and state. In perhaps the most graphic example of tensions between liberals and the Church hierarchy during the early Cold War, Eleanor Roosevelt accused Spellman of bigotry when he defended state taxes to support Catholic schools.[84] These kinds of clashes increased the climate of crisis that, in the eyes of the participants, seemed to surround the entire debate over euthanasia. Thus, if the verbal attacks on the Catholic Church by the ESA and organizations such as POAU sometimes overstepped the bounds of polite discussion, they did not differ substantially from the rhetoric emanating from Catholic quarters.

IV.

Catholic opposition to euthanasia dated back to the earliest public expressions of support for mercy killing at the time of the Bollinger baby case. As interest in the cause mounted in the 1930s, Catholic attacks intensified, reaching a fever peak at about the time of the founding of the ESA.[85] During World War II, Pope Pius XII spoke out against euthanasia on numerous occasions, most emphatically in a 1943 encyclical letter, in which he condemned the mercy killing of the mentally ill and the physically handicapped. With the end of the war, American Catholics increasingly drew connections between medical killing in the Third Reich and the euthanasia movement in the United States.[86]

Catholic readiness to link Nazism and the euthanasia movement drew ESA warhorse Charles Francis Potter back into the fray. In late 1946 Monsignor Robert E. McCormick, presiding justice of the Archdiocese of New York's ecclesiastical tribunal, attacked the ESA for seeking to introduce involuntary euthanasia once it had managed to get elective mercy killing legalized. Relying on the "wedge" argument, McCormick equated the ESA's aims and Nazi crimes. Potter counterattacked, saying that euthanasia could hardly be murder when it was practiced with "mercy aforethought," not malice. He also drew on the separation of church and state theory to insist that no church in America had the right to determine what was morally correct for all Americans. As he had done on more than one occasion, he gleefully pointed out that Thomas More, canonized by the Vatican in 1935, had depicted a society that permitted euthanasia in his *Utopia* of 1516. In this rough and tumble exchange of candid viewpoints with McCormick, Potter gave as good as he got. But any rhetorical victories he scored must have been tempered by the private realization that the Catholic "wedge" argument had a grain of truth to it.[87]

Battle between Catholics and the ESA was truly joined in 1949 over the petition of the Protestant and Jewish clergymen in defense of voluntary euthanasia and the ESA's campaign to introduce a euthanasia bill in the New York State assembly. Supporting the Roman Catholic Church was the American Council of Christian Churches with its fifteen separate denominations and a million and a half members, and the General Convention of the Protestant Episcopal Church. When, in 1950, the World Medical Association branded euthanasia as "contrary to public interest and to medical and ethical principles" under any circumstances, Cardinal Spellman rejoiced that the organization had affirmed the commandment "thou shalt not kill."[88]

Catholic objections to euthanasia in the 1930s and 1940s included traditional Church teaching about pain and suffering. Pain was due to the human condition of sin. Just as Christ had suffered a painful death, Catholics were enjoined to follow his example, thereby performing penance and acquiring the qualities of compassion. In that sense, suffering from "the mystical beauty of pain" was "a blessing in disguise," an opportunity to reconcile oneself with God rather than a curse.[89] Life was a gift from God and was therefore sacred. Those who committed suicide or euthanasia were flouting the responsibilities that accompanied this divine gift. Human beings were not free to do what they pleased with this gift. Thus, according to Catholic doctrine, euthanasia was an act of defiance and rebellion against God.[90]

Catholics also opposed euthanasia between the Depression and the end of the Cold War because they viewed it as a logical by-product of totalitarian politics.[91] This theory became an emphatic theme after World War II as anticommunism gathered momentum and news of Nazi atrocities broke. To Catholics, Nazi and Stalinist crimes were convincing confirmation of the Church's "wedge" argument, articulated as early as 1907 by Baltimore's James Cardinal Gibbons. Catholic critics contended that the legalization of euthanasia was symptomatic of a philosophy of "materialism" and "state absolutism," most evident in regimes such as Nazi Germany and Stalinist Russia. As one heated letter writer told the ESA in 1958, "I suggest you change your organization's name to Euthanasia Society of Communists, Inc. It seems your aim is more in line with communistic thinking than with a country such as ours. [Communists] don't believe in God and it seems you agree with them."[92] Materialism and "state absolutism" allegedly led to an erosion of the belief in the sanctity of individual human life and the willingness to believe that some lives were not worth living. Once this erosion began to take to place, Catholics charged, abuses would inevitably arise. Terminally ill patients might well be browbeaten into agreeing to euthanasia by friends or relatives who stood to benefit. Even worse, for economic and social reasons the state might decide it had the right to terminate the lives of individual citizens it deemed disposable. American Catholics pointed out how Germans had paid a fearsome price by tolerating the public advocacy of euthanasia in the first place.[93]

The quarrel between the ESA and the Catholic Church in America revealed that at the heart of their disagreement was a clash between two widely different moral and political philosophies. The Catholic Church held to a nonsecular view of the "quality of life." For Catholics, euthanasia was only one of several medical practices that, if accepted, would topple the entire edifice of Judeo-Christian morality. Like abortion, contraception, eugenic sterilization, and artificial insemination, euthanasia represented a repudiation of the sanctity of life and the inherent worth of each human being. When such values are compromised, Catholic leaders agreed, state tyranny is the result. In the wake of World War II, Catholic opponents of euthanasia felt history had proved them right.

In one sense, the Catholic interpretation of euthanasia was not all that different from that of euthanasia advocates. Both sides viewed eugenics, birth control, and euthanasia as kindred causes that were all part of a single project. Where they differed was in the fervent belief of euthanasia proponents that such a project, far from being a reason to worry, would instead lead to the emancipation of human beings. Euthanasia defenders believed wholeheartedly that legalizing euthanasia was, like the decriminalization of birth control, an important step toward the emergence of a new kind of citizen prepared to exercise his or her natural freedom—a citizen eminently equipped to resist the forces they believed threatened American democracy in the postwar era. Catholic and conservative Protestant success in thwarting these achievements only made the leaders of the euthanasia movement more convinced that these menacing forces had to be defeated if democracy was to survive. How to defeat them, however, amid the conservative cultural climate of the 1950s, remained a baffling and frustrating mystery.

V.

The 1940s and 1950s were a time of high expectations and incontestable accomplishments for the euthanasia movement, but they were also years of setbacks and grave disappointments. The movement had made "rapid progress in two decades," Potter told *Newsweek* magazine in 1958.[94] In 1952 the ESA had petitioned the Human Rights Commission of the United Nations to declare the right to die a basic human right for people dying of an incurable disease. The petition bore the signatures of over 2,500 prominent individuals from the United States and Great Britain. Although the United Nations did not adopt the request, the entire gesture symbolized the growing acceptance of euthanasia among the educated elites on both sides of the Atlantic. All that stood in the ESA's way were "old-fashioned religious hangovers," Potter declared.[95]

But Potter's optimism rang hollow in the 1950s. By then, few euthanasia advocates seriously expected to see euthanasia legalized in their lifetimes.[96] When an opinion poll in 1950 asked Americans whether they approved of allowing physicians by law to end incurably ill patients' lives by painless means if they and their families requested it, only 36 percent answered "yes," approximately 10 percent less than in the late 1930s.[97] In 1950, the 500,000-member World Medical Association voted to recommend to all national medical associations that euthanasia be condemned "under any circumstances."[98] The Catholic, Presbyterian, Episcopal, and fundamentalist churches were similarly united against the ESA.

Indeed, as early as 1951, Eleanor Dwight Jones was openly bemoaning that interest in euthanasia was waning.[99] To Jones, the public attention span was frustratingly short when it came to euthanasia, and this absence of sustained interest hindered the ESA's effectiveness. The society had never been a large operation and, as the 1950s wore on, its energies dissipated. By 1958, it still could not afford any full-time staff, nor could it afford to keep its Manhattan office (described by an ESA board member as "really a glorified broom closet") open all day, Monday to Friday.[100] Its budget was a meager $4,000 per year, and its sparsely attended meetings were usually held in the New York City apartment of Alice Naumburg Proskauer, a fervent but aged euthanasia activist.[101] As time went on, original friends and allies of the euthanasia movement passed away, a perennial problem for a cause that tended to attract elderly rather than youthful persons who were less worried about their mortality. Another sign that the movement needed an infusion of young blood was Charles Potter's return to the presidency in the early 1960s, just before he died. The death in 1954 of VELS founder C. Killick Millard was also a serious blow to the ESA, which had relied on his advice and eagerness to cooperate on international projects. The addition of educated, professional young people remained unlikely as long as organized medicine and most churches rejected euthanasia.

By the end of the 1950s, then, the ESA and its supporters had to face the fact that Americans were solidly opposed to the legalization of euthanasia.[102] Many Americans took a permissive attitude when individuals such as Hermann Sander helped terminally ill patients die from compassionate motives, but the majority of Americans drew a firm line between that sort of action and its decriminalization. The consensus was that it was better that all forms of physician-administered euthanasia remain illegal, with the threat of persecution serving as a deterrent. While this struck some as hypocritical (or worse), others were willing to live with this untidy compromise.

What few on either side of the debate realized during the 1950s, however, was that the times were about to change in dramatic ways. New attitudes, ideas, and medical technology would combine in the 1960s to alter the cultural landscape fundamentally. Disease, death, and dying quickly became some of the most consistently discussed and debated subjects in American public life. A new openness about euthanasia made it easier for advocates to broach the subject as a humane policy reform.

Although initially caught unprepared by these changes, the ESA would redefine itself in the 1960s and 1970s in an attempt to reconcile the long-standing objectives of the euthanasia movement with a revolutionary cultural climate stressing personal fulfillment and individual empowerment. By the 1980s the ESA's efforts would be largely successful, but the cost in unity was high. The process of adaptation to altered cultural and political attitudes bred factionalism and dissent among supporters of the right to die. The irony is that, just when unprecedented sympathy for euthanasia began to swell, the movement itself lost the cohesiveness it had tended to enjoy when it was embattled, small-scale, and socially elite. Then, it mattered little what intentions had inspired people to support euthanasia. Everyone seemingly shared a belief in the need to legalize active euthanasia, regardless of motive.

As the twentieth century neared its end, personal autonomy in death and dying became major popular concerns in American society, and the euthanasia movement gained adherents by the tens of thousands. But activists, who had once thought the issue was simple, learned to their dismay that winning grassroots support also led to disunity. Many converts to the cause were satisfied with the right to passive euthanasia, or the right to refuse unwanted treatment, but leery about active euthanasia. Euthanasia advocates had to acknowledge by the end of the twentieth century that the struggle to gain popular and political support for a right to die was proving to be much more difficult than anyone had imagined decades earlier.

4

Riding a Great Wave, 1960–1975

Few predicted it, but euthanasia suddenly burst onto the national scene in the 1960s and 1970s as an issue of sustained public interest. Under the shadow of nuclear war, in the wake of the thalidomide tragedy, amid a demoralizing war in southeast Asia, and in response to the aging of the U.S. population and the mounting use of life-prolonging medical technology, Americans became increasingly obsessed with death and terminal illness as experiences that deserved detailed study and discussion.[1] As a national dialogue on dying spread, the idea of death with minimal pain and loss of individual dignity grew popular. Thanks to the rising public interest in the concepts of patient autonomy and individual rights, euthanasia ceased being interpreted as a predominantly social or biological matter and was largely transformed into a personal issue. Increasingly it was viewed as a civil liberty, a freedom *from* interference in one's personal life, rather than a legal practice monitored (and possibly applied) by the state. Privacy became the keyword of the new, revitalized euthanasia movement, and the term "euthanasia" was steadily replaced by the phrase "the right to die."

This change helped to break the stalemate reached by the 1950s when euthanasia was chiefly defined in terms of the deliberate killing of terminally ill patients, and when discussion of euthanasia was hopelessly polarized. Ironically and unexpectedly, impetus for change came from Pope Pius XII, who, in 1957, announced that passive euthanasia was permissible, that patients could refuse extraordinary treatment to prolong their lives without violating Christian teaching. In a single stroke, the Pope helped to alter the terrain beneath the entire debate over euthanasia, making a constructive dialogue possible among those concerned about medical care for the dying and ending the standoff between the ESA and its opponents in the 1940s and 1950s.

But with the disappearance of the familiar fault lines between euthanasia advocates and their opponents, the old unity of the euthanasia movement began to dissolve as various groups advanced their own interpretations of the right to die. Gone were the customary eugenic justifications for mercy killing and the proposals for state-run euthanasia programs. To many Americans, euthanasia came to mean the right to refuse treatment. However, social and economic justifications for euthanasia did not disappear—a symptom of the mixed signals emitted by the 1960s counterculture—nor did the illiberal and elitist tendencies, stretching back to the Progressive era, which historically have characterized the campaign to legalize euthanasia.

I.

It was a pope, of all people, who truly revolutionized the national discussion over the right to die. On 24 February 1957 Pope Pius XII spoke to an international gathering of anesthesiologists and, while upholding traditional Catholic opposition to mercy killing, added that there was no reason that dying persons should endure unusual pain. Physicians, he stated, were permitted to use pain relievers even if they shortened a dying patient's life, though doctors should never administer pain-killing drugs against someone's will or with the intention of killing a patient. Christians were still encouraged to accept physical suffering as heroic imitation of Christ's passion on the Cross, but the Pope declared that dying patients were under no obligation to accept extraordinary medical treatment simply to extend their lives.[2]

The Pope's announcement in favor of passive (not active) voluntary euthanasia caught euthanasia proponents off guard. Since the ESA's inception, its leadership had crafted its message to the American public in terms of legalizing voluntary, active euthanasia. Euthanasia advocates had tended to ignore the issue of withdrawal of medical treatment for consenting, dying adults. Well into the 1950s, the ESA still included a sizable number of eugenically inclined members who were more interested in medical mercy killing. While figures such as Charles Potter and Eleanor Dwight Jones did not ignore the personal and humane virtues of individual choice-in-dying, they usually conflated these considerations with factors such as the savings to taxpayers and the emotional relief for friends and relatives. They appeared almost oblivious to what after the 1960s would become the swelling popular demand for an individual's right to refuse unwanted medical treatment. Hamstrung by their simultaneous commitments to birth control, eugenics, and population control, they seemed unable to conceptualize the right to refuse treatment as a purely humane step toward meeting the personal needs of terminally ill Americans. Both the Pope's address and the cultural changes of the 1960s compelled them to rethink their entire way of viewing euthanasia.

From the Catholic perspective, the Pope's gesture was brilliant strategy. Pius had been briefed extensively by his close friend, New York City's Francis Cardinal Spellman, a warhorse in the Church's battles with the ESA and Protestants and Other Americans United for the Separation of Church and State (POAU). Spellman was politically astute and, although a stern moralist, on a few topics was refreshingly open to new ideas.[3] He knew as much as anyone in the Church that the times and attitudes of Americans were changing, notably American Catholics whose misgivings about Church teaching on sex and contraception would be more evident in the 1960s. Spellman did not want to budge on sexual teachings, but on the ethics of palliative care he was more flexible.[4] Life-sustaining medical technology was making bedside decision-making more and more complex. Simply continuing to advocate a total ban on all forms of euthanasia was bound to be viewed as obstructionist and likely to discredit the Church in the long run. Conceding the right to refuse futile medical treatment might checkmate the ESA-led movement in favor of active euthanasia by raising questions about whether the latter was even necessary. Such a strategy might pressure euthanasia proponents to put their campaign in favor of active euthanasia on hold, which is precisely what they did.

In taking the advice of Cardinal Spellman, Pope Pius XII was also reacting to the first signs that philosophers and legal theorists were studying euthanasia. One of the weaknesses of the euthanasia movement up to the 1950s was that, while there had been polemics aplenty, no philosopher had attempted a systematic defense of euthanasia as an integral part of an overall revision of medical ethics. Charles Potter had been defending euthanasia since the 1930s, but like his colleagues in the movement, he had written little that could serve as a sophisticated philosophical justification of mercy killing.

When Potter died in 1962, theologian Joseph Fletcher assumed Potter's unofficial title as the chief philosopher of the euthanasia movement. By then, Fletcher's 1954 book *Medicine and Morals* had become a best seller and had almost single-handedly launched the discipline of biomedical ethics, ending the dominance practicing physicians had exercised for years over bedside decision-making in medicine.[5] Fletcher introduced the highly influential theory of "situational ethics," which stated that there were no absolute moral standards that guided medical treatment. The solution to any health-related dilemma depended solely on the particular circumstances surrounding a patient's condition.[6] The wide readership of *Medicine and Morals* and Fletcher's other books testified to the success he enjoyed between the 1950s and his death in 1991 breaking down barriers to the acceptance of euthanasia.

Fletcher, born in 1905 in Newark, New Jersey, ranks with Potter, Jones, Jack Kevorkian, and Hemlock Society co-founder Derek Humphry as the people who did the most for the right-to-die movement in twentieth-century America.[7] Although he wrote on a variety of biomedical issues, Fletcher was most interested in euthanasia, devoting the bulk of his last thirty years to the cause. Like so many others in the movement, Fletcher supported euthanasia—what he often called "death control"—because he saw it as a kindred cause to birth control and reproductive rights for women. "Death control, like birth control," he stated, "is a matter of human dignity. Without it persons become puppets."[8]

What marked him as a critical figure in the history of the euthanasia movement was the way he tried to distance himself from much of the social Darwinism that had punctuated earlier, eugenically oriented justifications of mercy killing. Instead, Fletcher fashioned a

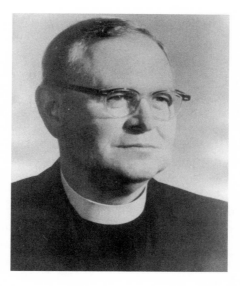

Joseph Fletcher. *Social Welfare History Archives, University of Minnesota.*

new rationale for euthanasia based primarily on the notion of patient autonomy. Fletcher's emphasis on what he called "the *personal*
dimensions of morality in medical care" helped to forge a new alli-
ance in the 1960s and 1970s between supporters of euthanasia and
those who supported women's right to abortion.[9]

An Episcopal minister, Fletcher in 1936 began pastoral counseling
of patients in homes and hospitals while teaching Christian ethics
at the Episcopal Theological School in Cambridge, Massachusetts. It
was his clinical experience dealing with the terminally ill that stimulated his interest in euthanasia, but from the beginning Fletcher
was temperamentally and intellectually disposed to embrace iconoclastic causes that stressed emancipation from traditional values. His
involvement in organizations such as the American Birth Control
League and the American Civil Liberties Union (ACLU) reflected
this tendency. Long before the family planning movement began
discussing a woman's right to terminate a pregnancy, Fletcher was
defending abortion. Twice beaten unconscious while lecturing in the
South for the Southern Tenants Farmers' Union, he became a member of the Soviet-American Friendship Society and the World Peace
Council after World War II, drawing the ire of Senator Joseph Mc-
Carthy, who called Fletcher "the Red Churchman." These experi-

ences made him a natural ally of the ESA in its battles with the Roman Catholic Church in the forties and fifties. In 1959 he denounced the "authoritarianism" of Catholicism as "alien to our American life and thought where cultural and religious pluralism is the most vital principle."[10] In fact, in the early 1940s, well before he became a target of McCarthyism, Fletcher and his friend Margaret Sanger had joined the ESA.[11]

In *Morals and Medicine*, Fletcher rehearsed some of Potter's old justifications for euthanasia. Why did society not accept euthanasia when it accepted war and capital punishment as excusable types of killing? Fletcher asked. Similarly, he interpreted the Sixth Commandment to mean "thou shalt do no murder," rather than "thou shalt not kill." As an ethicist, he rejected "naturalism" as a rationale for euthanasia and instead stressed freedom to choose for people whose "integrity [was] threatened by disintegration." Recalling the views of Felix Adler, Fletcher argued that "the principles of personal morality warn us not to make physical phenomena, unmitigated by human freedom, the center of life's meaning."[12]

Fletcher's rejection of naturalism as a basis for medical ethics had a powerful appeal in a day and age when social scientists were condemning eugenics and stressing "culture" over biology.[13] But his antinaturalism was far from complete. Fletcher quoted approvingly earlier euthanasia proponents such as Potter, Abraham Wolbarst, and Charlotte Perkins Gilman, who had expressed social Darwinist opinions in the past. At the same time he cited S. J. Holmes, a eugenicist and member of the ESA's advisory council, who in his *Life and Morals* (1948) had argued that morals *should* be based on "naturalistic" and "biological concepts."[14]

Fletcher's spirited defense of eugenic sterilization in *Morals and Medicine* also cast a shadow over his insistence that he sought only "private choice" in euthanasia. In 1962 Fletcher became president of the Human Betterment Association of America (HBAA), the new name chosen in 1950 for Marian Olden's Birthright, Inc., which endorsed voluntary sterilization (vasectomy or tubal ligation, but not castration) as both a family planning and population control technique.[15] Like so many members of the HBAA, Fletcher also recommended involuntary sterilization as a means of curbing the fertility of the mentally handicapped. As he declared in 1954, the "unborn" enjoyed a "complete *birthright* of a sound mind in a sound body," and this justified compulsory sterilization. "The interest of the public welfare" and the very "spiritual nature" of the individual permitted it. Even punitive sterilization of criminals was "ethically sound," according to Fletcher.[16]

Such reasoning undermined Fletcher's claim to defend only voluntary euthanasia. If the mentally handicapped and criminals should be forced to undergo sterilization for social reasons, then why should the state stop short of ordering the mercy killing of severely disabled individuals? If their hospitalization and medical treatment entailed high costs to the community, and if their quality of life appeared miserable in institutions, what prevented governments from taking measures to cut these costs in the name of "social justice" or "humanity"? Fletcher never answered these questions in *Morals and Medicine*.[17] By stressing that there was no rational or Christian reason to regard life as sacred, that painful dying or disability caused the personality to disintegrate, and that it was "indecent to go on living" under certain circumstances, Fletcher's ethical philosophy was something less than a denunciation of involuntary euthanasia. This became clearer in 1977 when he argued that "mercy killing" was justified for "an incorrigible 'human vegetable,' whether spontaneously functioning or artificially supported, [who] is progressively degraded while constantly eating up private or public financial resources in violation of the distributive justice owed to others." "The needs of others have a stronger claim upon us morally" than those of such a patient, he concluded. Little wonder that critics charged that his support for elective euthanasia was merely a tactic designed to acclimatize public opinion to the idea of mercy killing without consent.[18]

In later years, Fletcher would continue to play a prominent role in the right-to-die campaign, but in the meantime his *Morals and Medicine* sparked a lively debate. Few agreed with Fletcher, one exception being philosopher and ESA member Horace Kallen, who echoed Fletcher's point that elective euthanasia was not murder. "Safeguarding a person's right to die," Kallen contended, "when and as he chooses, so long as the exercise of this right works no violence on the rights of others, seems to me a proper function for the laws of a free society."[19] Paul Ramsey, professor of religion at Princeton University, was less enthusiastic than Kallen, deploring Fletcher's willingness to allow the state or medical profession to enter "the killing business."[20]

Fletcher's book inspired legal scholars to join the debate over euthanasia. While some acknowledged that the law regarding mercy killings had its problems, and that euthanasia ought to be seen as a lesser type of homicide, they were reluctant to make it legal lest it devalue human life. One Northwestern University legal scholar, employing Charles Potter's argument that public confidence in the law suffered when juries acquitted mercy killers, urged that "voluntary euthanasia administered by physicians" be decriminalized.[21] But the most important issue to emerge from the legal reaction to Fletcher's book was his affirmation of patient autonomy: that is, the right of patients to know the truth and their freedom to act on it as they saw fit. And the chief proponent of this viewpoint was the British legal scholar Glanville Williams.

Williams, like Fletcher, was hardly an impartial observer when it came to euthanasia. A member of both the ESA and the British Voluntary Euthanasia Legislation Society (VELS), Williams was already a convert to the cause when his *The Sanctity of Life and the Criminal Law* was published in 1957. Williams essentially repeated the argument made by anti-Catholic euthanasia advocates in the 1940s that the prohibition against euthanasia was defensible only on religious grounds and therefore did not apply to those who did not share such beliefs. To Williams, the main issue was "personal liberty."[22] Relying heavily on Fletcher, Williams repeated the standard reasons for rethinking euthanasia: that the Sixth Commandment really meant "thou shalt do no murder," not "thou shalt not kill"; that a merciful "assisted suicide" with the patient's consent was permissible if killing in war or the execution of criminals was allowed; and that denying suffering human beings the right to die was denying them the love and compassion Christians owed one another. People were "entitled to demand the release of death from hopeless and helpless pain," and physicians ought to be immune to prosecution if they helped willing individuals to die.[23]

However, again like Fletcher, Williams waffled on the subject of restricting euthanasia to consenting, dying adults. Besides granting that euthanasia could be legalized in cases of "incapacitating but non-painful affliction, such as paralysis," he also broached the topic of involuntary euthanasia in cases of senile dementia and "hopelessly defective infants." Williams conceded that putting senile people to death would never be permitted unless "generally accepted values" were overthrown, but then again, he did not seem terribly worried that this might happen. He had even fewer qualms about euthanasia for defective infants. As long as there was parental consent, Williams saw nothing wrong in infants "being done to death," as it could be justified on "eugenic" and "humanitarian" grounds. "[I]nfants cannot, like adults, feel anticipatory dread" of dying, he wrote, so putting them to death was not as cruel as many imagined. The litany of twentieth-century court cases involving parents mercy killing their handicapped children showed that "the legalization of euthanasia for handicapped children would simply bring the law into closer relation to its practical administration," because juries usually acquitted such parents.[24]

Williams's theory that euthanasia could be condemned only for religious reasons was attacked by Yale Kamisar, a University of Minnesota Law School professor, on the grounds that there were legitimate nonreligious objections to euthanasia.[25] Kamisar's criticism of Williams is as powerful today as it was in the 1950s. Euthanasia was unnecessary because doctors were getting better and better at controlling pain with medication. It was dangerous because physicians might misdiagnose an illness and thereby sway personal decisions to request euthanasia. Kamisar had few objections to voluntary euthanasia if all preconditions were strictly met. "But abstract propositions and carefully formed hypotheticals are one thing; specific proposals designed to cover everyday situations are something else again." The devil, in other words, was in the details, and any one law—no matter how safeguarded—was bound to lead to abuses. If suffering individuals were intent on suicide, it was better, he concluded, to take a "laissez-faire" attitude to the whole issue than pursue the enactment of a law "sanctioned by the state." Changing the law would be worse than leaving the law as it was.[26]

Kamisar subscribed to the "wedge" argument used by Catholics and other religious opponents of euthanasia, contending that the "legal machinery initially designed to kill those who are a nuisance to themselves may someday engulf those who are a nuisance to others."[27] Kamisar quoted at length from both ESA and VELS literature, which showed clear approval of involuntary as well as voluntary euthanasia. He also cited the Viennese-born psychiatrist Leo Alexander, who, after serving as consultant to the U.S. Office of the Chief Counsel for War Crimes at the Nuremberg Trials (1946–1947), argued that the horrors of the Holocaust could be traced to "small beginnings" before the Nazis took power in Germany.[28] Once individuals such as Karl Binding and Alfred Hoche started talking about lives "not worthy to be lived," it became permissible to refer to some people being "better off dead." Given the tiny size and strength of America's euthanasia movement in the 1950s, Kamisar admitted that it was unlikely that Nazi-like atrocities would happen in America, but the internment of Japanese-Americans during the Second World War showed "*it can happen here unless we darn well make sure that it does not* by adamantly holding the line, by swiftly snuffing out what are or might be small beginnings of what we do not want to happen here."[29]

Thus, by the end of the 1950s the arguments of people such as Kamisar, who linked euthanasia to the horrors of the Third Reich, put the euthanasia movement squarely on the defensive. The fact that Fletcher and Williams linked acceptance of euthanasia to approval of other such highly controversial policies as abortion and eugenic sterilization made their task of trying to win public opinion even more challenging. Juries might be sympathetic toward parents who ended the lives of their handicapped children, but that did not translate into any groundswell of opinion in favor of changing the laws regarding mercy killing.

The campaign for euthanasia was going so poorly by the early 1960s that even Joseph Fletcher recognized the need for a change of tactics. No one was better able to sniff the prevailing winds than Fletcher, and so he began to modify his approach to the issue in the short term, emphasizing the need to legalize passive euthanasia. He even proposed dropping the word "euthanasia" with its Nazi overtones, and replacing it with "dysthanasia," meaning "mercifully refusing to prolong the process of dying."[30] "Dysthanasia" never caught on, but it is a measure of the demoralization sweeping the euthanasia movement at the time that militants such as Fletcher were so willing to soften their message in the struggle to win the backing of Americans. In the 1970s Fletcher and other radicals would recover their confidence and start campaigning for active euthanasia, but his moderation in the 1960s was a signal that the battle over the legalization of euthanasia was not going well for his side.

II.

Fletcher's gnawing feeling that the drive to legalize euthanasia had stalled by the early 1960s was shared by numerous ESA members. ESA activities had virtually ground to a halt.[31] The volume of correspondence to and from the ESA declined to the point where many members were unsure whether it had disbanded.[32] In September 1962 only 325 memberships were paid up. Saddled with the reputation of advocating a "radical cause," the ESA found it difficult to attract funding. Magazines such as *Harper's* and the *Atlantic Monthly* refused to print ESA advertisements.[33] Mainstream opinion, which only a decade earlier had showed signs of shifting in favor of euthanasia, appeared distinctly unreceptive.

Any lingering hopes that a state legislature would pass a voluntary euthanasia bill were dashed in 1962 when, amid considerable media scrutiny, three ex-Nazis were indicted in Germany for their complicity in Hitler's euthanasia program.[34] Such news revived bad memories for the ESA of its tribulations in the late 1940s fending off accusations that it endorsed Nazi-like atrocities.[35] The chief effects of the unwanted publicity were to convince more and more ESA members that the organization's short-term future lay in trying to educate public opinion about death and dying before launching any further attempts to legalize mercy killing.

Changing public opinion first was the policy of choice for Pauline Taylor, lawyer and ESA president from 1962 to 1964.[36] Taylor, born in 1910, at one time had been a director of the American Birth Control League of America. In the late 1950s she and Sidney Rosoff, a tax lawyer, had sought to solve the ongoing financial troubles of the ESA by forming the separate Euthanasia Educational Fund (EEF) as a tax-exempt charitable organization, in the hopes of raising more revenue through donations, especially from the large foundations.[37] Although president for only two short years, Taylor also began the ESA's soul-searching process that led to a major shift in philosophy for the entire American euthanasia movement. She believed the ESA in the past had overemphasized the soundness of an individual's decision to have his or her life ended if terminally ill and in unbearable pain, and thought the movement had failed by not "adopt[ing] a position on the thorny subject of the treatment of patients beyond reasonable hope of recovery. . . . In this respect we are in the rear of the late Pope [Pius XII]." Taylor concluded that the time was ripe to follow the Pope's cue and begin convincing the public that letting someone die, instead of resorting to extreme measures, was both humane and ethically permissible. This plan appealed to the less militant members of the ESA who were not sure that the legalization of active euthanasia was what they really wanted, but it also appealed to the supporters of legalizing active euthanasia because it seemed to be the best strategy for preparing public opinion to accept their goals in the long run. By appealing to both groups, this strategy managed to keep the euthanasia movement united for another decade.[38]

Taylor's attempts to change the orientation of the euthanasia movement by discouraging overtreating of the terminally ill and de-emphasizing euthanasia legislation were taken up by the Unitarian minister Donald McKinney, who became president of the ESA in 1965. McKinney, whose crucial influence over the euthanasia movement would extend into the 1990s, succeeded the short-lived presidency of Presbyterian minister John Paul Jones, chairman of the board of the New York Civil Liberties Union, who had just died at the age of sixty-seven. Jones was someone who typified the affinity between the cause of euthanasia and Cold War, anti-McCarthyite liberalism, having been attacked (like Fletcher) as being soft on communism by the McCarthyites.[39] It was Jones who asked McKinney whether he would like to serve on the ESA's board, and at the very first board meeting McKinney attended he was offered its presidency.[40]

Once he became president, McKinney quickly put his own stamp on the ESA. Over the next two decades he would help to transform the euthanasia movement by leading a sizable faction opposed to active euthanasia or physician-assisted suicide. In the process he eventually concluded, in contrast to colleagues such as Joseph Fletcher, that there was a fundamental distinction between passive and active euthanasia. This point became a serious bone of contention that would divide the movement in the late 1970s. The shock waves were still being felt in the early twenty-first century.

McKinney was yet another example of the strong historical link between Unitarianism and the euthanasia movement. Born in 1927, he grew up in Bridgewater, Massachusetts, where his father was a Unitarian minister. Later he enrolled in Harvard Divinity School and decided there to follow his father's footsteps. His first post was as assistant to John Howland Lathrop, the minister at the First Unitarian Church in Brooklyn, New York, and himself a former ESA vice-president. Lathrop had been one of the first and best-known clergymen recruited by the ESA in its campaign to prove that there were no religious objections to euthanasia. McKinney succeeded Lathrop at the First Unitarian Church in 1957 and served as its senior minister until his retirement in 1992.[41]

McKinney was part of a new generation of activists entering the euthanasia movement in the 1960s, and this was reflected in his willingness to envisage a new direction for the ESA. When McKinney took over as president in 1965, the change in the ESA was almost immediately noticeable. As a relatively young thirty-eight-year-old, McKinney symbolized ESA hopes to interest America's youth on university and college campuses in euthanasia and dispel its image as an organization of elderly people obsessed by their own mortality.[42] McKinney and ESA secretary Katharine (Kay) Mali proceeded to build the ESA from a tiny operation into an organization with major cultural clout and an annual budget by the 1970s in the hundreds of thousands of dollars.[43]

Kay Mali followed much the same route as other women ESA members in their migrations to the euthanasia movement. A graduate of Bryn Mawr College, she was active for years in the family planning field as a one-time director of the American Birth Control League, and later Planned Parenthood of Manhattan and the Bronx. She joined the board of the ESA in 1955 and became president of the EEF in 1969 while McKinney recovered from hepatitis. She continued as president until her death by suicide in 1980 at the age of seventy-eight. Mali saw her involvement in family planning and euthanasia as different aspects of the same overall crusade to liberate Americans from traditional values and customs.[44]

Over the course of 1965, McKinney, Mali, and the ESA board forged a new statement of the ESA's purposes and goals. Gone were any references to legislative reform. Emphasis was placed on "education, research, and public dialogue" as means for "encourag[ing] full consideration of the ethical, legal and medical questions involved in an incurable sufferer's right to die, if he so petitions." To achieve this objective, the ESA formed a speakers' bureau and targeted institutions of higher education, especially graduate schools of theology, law, and medicine, as well as medical societies and other professional groups. The organization sponsored seminars for physicians, clergy, and medical students, exploring suicide, grief therapy, caring for the dying patient, educational courses on bereavement, and the like. ESA officials appeared on television and radio talk shows, and the movement received a big boost when entertainers Arthur Godfrey and Patricia Neal endorsed the right to die. Beginning in 1968, at the Carnegie International Endowment Center in New York City, the ESA also held annual conferences featuring prominent speakers, such as Lael Wertenbaker, author of the 1957 best-seller *Death of a Man*, the story of her husband's battle with cancer and ultimate suicide.[45] Overall, the new ESA called for a nationwide discussion of the full range of issues surrounding death and dying, and it encouraged the creation of state organizations and other local groups to pursue research and disseminate information.[46] Thanks to these initiatives, within a few short years, the ESA had been energized like never before.[47]

III.

The change in the ESA's fortunes would never have occurred had it not been for the sweeping changes America underwent, starting in the 1960s.[48] The temptation is to reduce the energization of the euthanasia movement to the important developments in medical, life-sustaining technology, as an understandable response to practical problems posed by instrumental changes in medical treatment. That is certainly part of the story. But the unprecedented receptiveness of the American people to euthanasia was due more to the cultural unrest of the 1960s than to changes in medical care. Public approval of euthanasia had been high in the 1930s, predating any wide use of major therapeutic interventions to keep patients alive. Popular revulsion toward life-sustaining medical methods was more a product of the broad antiestablishment attitudes of the sixties and seventies than a product of the technology itself.[49]

In the 1960s, against the backdrop of a steadily declining faith in the country's institutions, women, African-Americans, college students, Native Americans, and other groups staged strikes and protests against poverty, pollution, the Vietnam War, and racial and sexual discrimination. One strain of this countercultural ferment, evident in the struggle for reproductive rights for women, was individualistic, accentuating personal privacy and choice. Many reformers, believing that all individual Americans deserved the same civil rights, also sought to end segregation in the South by working across racial lines.

However, demands for self-determination and individual rights jostled awkwardly in the sixties with appeals to group rights and aggressive government measures to end injustice. Communitarian, public, and collectivist themes were evident in rock music concerts, hippie communes, "Black Power" separatism, and New Left "street theater" demonstrations. These elements helped to produce a cultural climate that tolerated some forms of violence and various extreme solutions to social problems. Environmentalists Paul Ehrlich and Garrett Hardin (later a member of the Santa Barbara chapter of the Hemlock Society) and groups such as Zero Population Growth stated that coercive measures might be necessary to control the population growth they claimed led to global pollution.[50] The legacy of the 1960s, so crucial for the subsequent fortunes of the euthanasia movement, was—like Progressivism before it—an uneasy mix of individualism and collectivism, authoritarian and liberationist elements, a brew that eventually began to worry some ESA activists such as Donald McKinney. The fear, as critics had warned since the days of Alexis de Tocqueville, was that the search for equality in democratic nations might lead to a "soft tyranny" that sanctioned state coercion in the name of social justice.[51]

These tensions became more obvious when, in the early 1970s, America's cultural climate turned sullen. Watergate, inflation, unemployment, defeat in Vietnam, the oil crisis, and the backlash against the Great Society reforms of the 1960s cumulatively undermined the country's confidence in its leadership and direction.[52] The malaise engendered by these trends and events sapped the diffuse optimism that had sustained the country since World War II and left Americans less sanguine about the power of science, medicine, and technology. As faith in progress fell, Americans became more willing to approve unconventional approaches to health and sickness, such as euthanasia.[53]

The malaise that gripped America in the 1970s deeply affected organized medicine. During its "golden age" in the first half of the twentieth century American medicine had enjoyed a "mandate" based on two premises: one, that the more medical care the public received the better off it was; and two, that medicine's practitioners, researchers, hospitals, and medical schools should be given the authority to run their own affairs as they saw fit. This mandate abruptly came to an end in the seventies.[54] Doctors' public esteem dropped from 72 to 57 percent between 1965 and 1973.[55] Criticism of medicine's greed, impersonality, resistance to reform, and overreliance on technology mounted during these years. Events such as the disaster caused by the sedative thalidomide, which, before it was withdrawn in 1961, caused hundreds of infants in Europe and Canada to be born with severe physical handicaps, convinced many that unregulated medicine was a threat to public health.[56]

Declining trust in medical science also derived from the fact that fewer and fewer people were dying from infectious diseases over the course of the first half of the twentieth century.[57] But as life expectancy rose steadily, and Americans lived longer lives after World War II, more and more people were exposed to mechanistic treatments for terminal illnesses, including respirators, artificial feeding, kidney dialysis, and organ transplants. In Joseph Fletcher's words, by the 1970s death had "changed its shape. . . . People are dying in hospitals now. . . . They die comatose and betubed and sedated and aerated and glucosed and *non compos mentis*. It has become a pretty ugly business."[58] Dehumanizing technologies, when combined with the "can-do" attitudes of many physicians, led countless Americans to believe doctors were prolonging rather than mitigating suffering.[59] This was reflected in a 1972 *Life* magazine survey of 41,000 readers, which showed that 91 percent believed a terminal patient should be permitted to refuse treatment that artificially extended life.[60]

One critic traced doctors' determination to see patient death as their failure to "the underlying bias of the technological mindset . . . that newer is better and that doing more must be better than doing less."[61] Historian Arnold Toynbee blamed it on the widespread belief that death itself was "un-American," and, as an affront to the political ethos of the nation, had to be fought relentlessly.[62] Whatever the cause, doctors were transformed into "strangers at the bedside," in David Rothman's words, and hospitals, once viewed as shining symbols of scientific medicine and public philanthropy, were perceived increasingly as cold and alienating places. Malpractice suits multiplied, self-medication and self-diagnosis spread, and medical schools scrambled to teach their students to be more sensitive and caring. In 1973 the American Medical Association adopted a "Patient's Bill of Rights," which recognized the right of patients to refuse treatment and be informed of all medical consequences. Many believed that these developments were steps in the right direction, but there was no discounting how they stemmed from the wider malaise that afflicted all of society. Escalating interest in euthanasia was another symptom of the popular perception that science and technology did not guarantee a better quality of life. Doing more for patients was not necessarily better than doing less.

Wide-ranging public disenchantment with organized medicine translated into a new, "postmodern" patient (in the words of historian Edward Shorter), someone who was defiant of medical authority, willing to experiment with alternative medicine, and increasingly anxious about his or her own health. The postmodern patient was especially distrustful of doctors' motives, skills, and claims to expertise, often supporting efforts to delegate health care to other practitioners. The postmodern patient was also more prone to interpret bodily sensations as signs of disease than patients of earlier generations. Postmodern patients were (and are) the ultimate consumers, receptive to a discourse that depicts the right to die as something patients can demand of their doctors in the same way they demand drug prescriptions when they are feeling depressed or stressed.[63]

The declining confidence in and mounting impatience with organized medicine was mirrored in American attitudes toward cancer, the disease most often associated with euthanasia. Between the late nineteenth century and the 1950s, American medical science had gone from one therapeutic success to another, discovering cures for a host of frightening diseases, including tuberculosis, syphilis, diphtheria, cholera, and the plague. The availability of blood and plasma for transfusions had dramatically improved the scope and effectiveness of surgery. The introduction of penicillin by the end of World War II and the announcement of the Salk vaccine for polio in 1955 convinced many Americans that a cure for cancer too was just around the corner.[64] The declaration of a "war on cancer" in 1971 sprang from the residual optimism surrounding these breakthroughs. But rather than being the first salvo in a victorious conquest of the "dread disease," the declaration of war on cancer was followed rapidly by a significant drop in public confidence that the scourge could be cured. After decades of great expectations that cancer would be licked, the mood of the country collapsed in the 1970s in the face of evidence that this war, even if victorious, would be exceedingly long and costly. Actually, between 1930 and 1960 five-year survival rates for cancer went from one in five to one in three, but Americans, though generally "doing better," were "feeling worse" about the future prospects for good health.[65] They were becoming increasingly skeptical about the cancer industry's ability to win the war against cancer. Patients' thoughts naturally began to shift to "self-deliverance," rather than waiting patiently for an iffy cure.

Suspicions about the efficacy and good intentions of America's medical profession were nowhere more evident than in the women's movement. The 1965 Supreme Court ruling in *Griswold v. Connecticut*, reversing an 1879 Connecticut anticontraception law and legalizing the sale of contraceptives, at first glance simply looked like the final victory after decades of birth control activism. Instead, by affirming a right to privacy implied in the Third, Fourth, and Fifth Amendments to the Constitution, the ruling sounded one of the foremost *leitmotifs* of the sixties' women's movement. It led in 1973 to *Roe v. Wade*, the Supreme Court ruling that legalized abortion, a decision also based on a woman's constitutional right to privacy and choice. The notion of a right to privacy seemed to capture the general ethos of the women's movement, aptly expressed in the best-selling *Our Bodies, Ourselves* (1973), a kind of self-help manual of women's health. In its pages and elsewhere, women demanded a franker, less authoritarian relationship to their doctors, objected to specific treatments (such as radical mastectomies) for women, protested the lack of women doctors in the profession, and sought to demystify organized medicine's claim to special knowledge about female physiology and psychology.[66] The women's movement spearheaded a countercultural campaign that urged women to learn more about their bodies as a way of defeating medical paternalism. "Health feminism," or "vaginal politics," spawned all-female gynecological clinics, rape crisis centers, and abortion counseling services across the nation.[67]

As this current within the women's movement gathered momentum in the early 1970s, however, the same tension between collective and individual rights that characterized the rest of the counterculture surfaced. What comes first: personal liberation or group solidarity? Individual autonomy or "a protective standard of inviolable differences"? In the area of reproductive politics, this was a particularly nettlesome matter. Where did one's right to choose end and society's right to protect its interests begin (as Joseph Fletcher phrased the question)? The same ambiguities dogged the euthanasia issue. In cases of terminal illness or chronic disability, what was more important: individual consent or the state's obligation to provide "humane" treatment? Exactly whose "right" was it to "pull the plug"? Despite the many signs that during the 1960s the nation had reached a revolutionary watershed in its history, consensual answers to these questions were as elusive then as they had been in the Progressive era.[68]

Feminist calls for the end of medical paternalism inevitably encompassed the topic of death and dying. As social activists toppled ages-old barriers between women and sexual and reproductive freedom, people began to demand that the taboo of silence surrounding death be similarly lifted. Such demands resonated with countless women. Like men, they were concerned about personal end-of-life circumstances and the possibility of losing their dignity during terminal illness. But their interest in euthanasia also derived from gendered, Victorian traditions that lasted well into the twentieth century. Professional nurses tended to be female, and women in general were expected to undertake the care of the sick and dying as a normal part of their nurturing role in the family. Similarly, just as some diseases afflicted women more than men, so women tended to live longer than men and thus had more opportunities to witness the death of loved ones. That also meant they, more than men, faced the prospect of dying alone and depending on strangers for their care.[69] As the personal stories of many women involved in the euthanasia movement attest, the experience of watching relatives, spouses, friends, or other patients die lingering deaths was heart-wrenching as well as consciousness-raising. In response, women struggled to take back death from the (largely male) medical profession, much as they had sought to do for sex, birth, and reproduction. They tended to be particularly sympathetic toward efforts to reduce pain and discomfort for the dying, viewing it as an additional act of emancipation from what Margaret Sanger had called "biological slavery."[70]

Understandably, then as the twentieth century drew to a close, women formed majorities in right-to-die groups, but most were not fire-breathing radicals. They were usually "affluent white women with gray hair . . . the sort of community-minded grandmothers who never littered, never stole anyone's parking place, and always returned their library books on time."[71] As one euthanasia activist put it, the typical member of a right-to-die group was "the little old Ohio lady in tennis shoes."[72]

The demystification of death at the hands of feminists was part of a wider trend in American culture, which saw death cease to be regarded as a taboo topic. "Nothing's sacred anymore," uttered a

Michigan internist in 1976. "First it was sex, and now it's death and dying. If the 1960s were the era of sexual revolution, the 1970s are the age of thanatology."[73] A "death craze" swept the country as books, magazines, radio, and television seemed fixated on the issue in the 1960s and 1970s.[74] Death had definitely come "out of the closet."[75]

Interest in death and dying led to the founding in 1969 of the Hastings Center, headed by Daniel Callahan, effectively launching the discipline of bioethics. Universities and medical schools taught courses and held seminars on death and dying. After 1970, books on death appeared at the rate of about one per month.[76] Movies such as *Brian's Song*, *I Never Sang for My Father*, and *They Shoot Horses, Don't They?* confirmed that death was a major theme in American culture. "Death is the most important question of our time," declared psychiatrist Robert Jay Lifton.[77] With data showing that suicide rates for Americans under the age of thirty-five had risen sharply since the end of World War II, there seemed to be even more reason to end "the silence about death."[78]

A major event that helped to end such "silence" occurred over three days in August 1972, when the U.S. Senate Special Commission on Aging (SCA) held hearings on "death with dignity." The SCA hearings, chaired by Senator Frank Church, proved to be a superb opportunity for professionals and laypeople to discuss a range of issues relating to aging and terminal illness, including the evolving doctor-patient relationship and the difficulties about defining death itself. Overall, the hearings showed that Americans were becoming increasingly unhappy about "the brutal irony of medical miracles," which extended the dying process only to diminish patient dignity and quality of life.[79] Church insisted that the hearings were not about euthanasia, but try as he might, he could not keep the subject from surfacing, a strong indication of the growing difficulties separating "death with dignity" from aid in dying.[80]

The hearings were also noteworthy because prominent physicians, including Henry K. Beecher, confessed that they had ceased life-sustaining treatment so some of their patients could die.[81] Henry Beecher's notoriety also stemmed from his efforts during these years to establish the revolutionary definition of brain death, replacing the traditional definition based on heart-lung failure. Beecher had chaired the Ad Hoc Committee of the Harvard Medical School to Examine the Definition of Brain Death. The committee's 1968 report proposed that physicians use a set of criteria to determine whether a patient had suffered permanent loss of all brain functions. Beecher had hoped the new definition would allay public suspicions that doctors, in their haste to harvest organs for transplantation, were "ghouls hovering over an accident victim with long knives unsheathed, waiting to take out his organs."[82] His hopes of co-opting such antiprofessional sentiments were never realized completely, but the committee's new definition of brain death did prove successful when it was depicted as a means of preventing aggressive doctors from using machinery to extend the dying process unnecessarily. Those who feared being hooked up to respirators with no vital signs of brain activity were reassured by the Harvard criteria, hardly surprising given that Beecher and Joseph Fletcher were good friends, and Beecher admired Fletcher's theory of situation ethics.[83]

Yet another landmark of the "age of thanatology" was Elisabeth Kübler-Ross's *On Death and Dying* (1969), which by 1976 had sold over a million copies. Although Kübler-Ross's theory about death being a five-step process ultimately failed to convince many ethicists, her description of dying as more "lonely, mechanical, and dehumanized" than in the past made her one of the most important opinion makers of her generation. "We live in a very peculiar, death-denying society," she told Senator Church's committee in 1972. "We isolate both the dying and the old, and it serves a purpose, I guess. They are reminders of our own mortality."[84]

Many hailed this "rediscovery of death" as a salutary development. But others questioned whether the subject of dying was being "worked to death." One critic in 1975 suggested society, instead of becoming more "open" about death, had simply become more "talkative." Many discussions about death were characterized by refreshing candor, but rather than leading to realistic and sober approaches to the topic, they seemed to foster little more than "foreboding" and "disenchantment."[85]

Often hidden beneath the frankness was the revolutionary fact that the nineteenth-century theory that redemption for dying people meant enduring their suffering simply was no longer fashionable. By the late twentieth century, dying increasingly meant a process in which patients obtained gratification through the consumption of specific products and services, but how to measure consumer gratification during dying was a question often overlooked by thanatologists. Too, there was a worrisome undercurrent running through much of the national debate over death. The popularity of Kübler-Ross's model masked a growing "irritation at those dying individuals who refused the new orthodoxy of the 'good death,' " who failed to conform and embrace the "happy death." In the fanfare surrounding new theories of death, many lost sight of the distinction between the prescriptive and the normative, equating what *ought* to be done with what *is* actually done.[86] The best of intentions ran the perilous risk of moving society toward consequences of which it was only dimly aware.

Thus, as historian Peter Filene has noted, by obsessing over death in the sixties and seventies, Americans had less demystified the topic than projected onto it "the confusions of modern culture." Death was now open to a wide range of interpretations, a situation that activists such as Joseph Fletcher would seek to exploit as the 1970s wore on. Initially, this absence of consensus on death and dying looked liberating and invited debate and discussion. Beneath the veneer of liberation, however, were mixed signals that continued to shape the various ways Americans defined euthanasia.[87]

IV.

Whether driven by the desire for self-actualization or mere narcissism, the attention paid to death strengthened America's "rights culture," and one of this trend's casualties was the word "euthanasia" itself. Tainted by its association with Nazism, its popularity among ESA members plummeted throughout the 1960s, culminating in two important name changes. In 1974, the Euthanasia Society of America became the Society for the Right to Die (SRD), and in 1977 the Euthanasia Educational Fund (having changed its name to the Euthanasia Educational Council in 1972) became Concern for Dying (CFD). In the 1940s and 1950s, the term "euthanasia" had become synonymous with mercy killing in the eyes of public opinion, or just plain killing. Instead of euthanasia in the sense of putting someone to death, the ESA's "new program" in the 1960s highlighted "the right to die" as "a human right, almost a civil liberty." Advocates increasingly preferred the right to die as the slogan for the movement, evoking the image of a "choice between prolonged suffering from terminal illness or a peaceful and dignified death."[88] Exercising one's right to die "in dignity" was also a throwback to the pre-twentieth-century meaning of euthanasia as an "easy death," or being allowed to die in peace and comfort when all efforts had proven futile. The big difference between the two eras, however, was that many Americans after the 1960s viewed a good death less as a blessing and more as a constitutional right.[89]

The leadership of the ESA in the 1960s was fully conscious that in striking out in such new directions it was "caught up in an awesomely large revolution," as Donald McKinney put it.[90] By pointing its message toward the country's college students it was hoping to ride the crest of a "great wave" of youthful protest sweeping the nation.[91] The emphasis on euthanasia as a "right to die" and a "choice" not to suffer needlessly fit the prevailing belief of the late 1960s that "my body is my own," and that no one—notably a doctor—should dictate how someone else experienced dying. Euthanasia became firmly associated with "human dignity" and personal autonomy. As an ESA official stated in 1966, attitudes toward death were changing "in an age when a lot of the old absolutes aren't so absolute anymore. Men and women are demanding the right to determine their own futures."[92] Or, as one Unitarian minister wrote in 1970, euthanasia was "a basic civil right," similar to the right to an abortion. "[G]overnment has the right to protect and define it only, but not the right to forbid it. It should be legally available to all competent persons, and government has no more right to confine it to suffering persons and deadly diseases than it has to curb freedom of religion."[93] In the coming years, numerous euthanasia proponents agreed that such a "civil rights" approach might win much-needed support for their cause among certain segments of American society.

Nothing demonstrated more how far the new ESA, with its celebration of self-determination, was distancing itself from the old ESA than the way its executive handled an invitation to participate in a conference on population control in 1965. Prior to this date the ESA would have jumped at such an opportunity to gain needed publicity and build coalitions with other reform groups. Ordinarily, ESA representatives would have been honored to share the podium with a roster of speakers that included such well-known champions of liberationist causes as Alan Guttmacher, president of Planned Parenthood Federation of America (and ESA board member); John Rock, codiscoverer of the first oral contraceptive pill; and Robert E. Hall, president of the Association for Humane Abortion. But the presence of Frederick Osborn, secretary-treasurer of the American

Eugenics Society, and a session dedicated to eugenics in Japan convinced the ESA to decline the invitation. Twenty years earlier, the ESA board would have hardly feared association with eugenics; in 1965, with eugenics gradually becoming a "dirty word" in the social and biological sciences, McKinney and Mali understandably chose not to attend.[94] The conference's willingness to entertain "compulsory" or legislative solutions to world population growth, such as nonelective sterilization, could not have been more alien to the ESA's affirmation of euthanasia in the sixties as an individual civil right.[95]

As fashionable as the ESA's "rights" message was in the 1960s, it was not entirely new; to a degree, the rest of the country was merely catching up to what many of the society's supporters, such as Charles Potter and Horace Kallen, had been preaching for years. The dovetailing of the ESA's retooled image and America's cultural revolution signaled the mounting resonance of the Humanist philosophy that dated back to the 1930s when Potter, his Unitarian allies, and some of the liberal clergymen who belonged to POAU were advocating euthanasia as a form of democratic citizenship in action. This curious mix of old and new radicalism was not only characteristic of the 1960s countercultural climate; it was true of the euthanasia movement itself. To old-timers in the movement such as Joseph Fletcher, it must have looked as if Americans were finally waking up to his call for discarding the old taboos and constructing an entirely new code of medical ethics.

In the meantime, the ESA created the Euthanasia Educational Fund, a separate organization, entirely educational in nature and therefore tax exempt. The ESA itself soon lapsed into virtual inaction, its legislative agenda postponed. The ESA's revival in 1974 as the Society for the Right to Die would indicate that interest in legislative reform was then rekindling, and it would trigger bitter, internecine conflicts within the movement over the next fifteen years.

The other crucial development in the history of the euthanasia movement in the 1960s was the introduction of the "living will." The living will, essentially capturing the spirit of Pope Pius XII's 1957 *allocutio,* is a document that states in advance a patient's request to discontinue treatment that simply prolongs life when the patient is dying and unable to make the decision. What the living will meant for the euthanasia movement was expressed by an ESA official in 1971, when she declared the living will is the keystone of a passive euthanasia which insists on your right to die with dignity with no heroic measures to keep you alive and prolong the days and hours of your dying. . . . In the early days of the Euthanasia Society we tried for legislation and got thousands of names on petitions to the legislature, but we found it needed more than that. It needed a strong public opinion and judging from the upsurge of interest in the subject in the past year, we think we are making some headway.[96]

The idea of the living will had actually surfaced in ESA circles as early as 1949, but at that time the concept of passive euthanasia was either ignored or dismissed as tangential to the movement's real objectives.[97] Less than twenty years later, however, a Chicago human rights lawyer named Luis Kutner reintroduced the idea, and this time it caught fire. An EEF committee drafted a model living will and then printed 5,000 copies in 1969. Within nine months, all 5,000 copies had been distributed.[98]

The concept behind the living will ideally suited the shifting American cultural climate of the 1960s and 1970s with its growing emphasis on the right to privacy and the emancipation of patients from impersonal, alienating, and technocratic professions and institutions. Although it was not yet legally binding, the living will appeared to give individuals back a measure of personal control over their own lives. Its rapid popularization was chiefly responsible for the EEF's astonishing growth in a few short years. By 1978, about three million living wills had been distributed by the EEF, thanks immeasurably to its promotion by advice columnist "Dear Abby" (Abigail Van Buren).[99] Because so many who requested a living will ended up joining and donating to the EEF, by 1975 it could claim some 70,000 members, a far cry from its several hundred supporters in the early 1960s. Its annual budget grew from $12,000 to over $400,000 in the ten years after 1967, and the organization's *Bulletin* reached over 100,000 people. By the late 1970s the organization's fiscal woes were a thing of the past. All that was left to decide was how to spend the money that flowed into the EEF's coffers. Predictably, this soon proved to be a highly divisive issue.

In 1976, California became the first state to recognize the living will. Within a year seven other states had enacted analogous statutes, and by 1986 all but eleven states had done the same. The living will's remarkable success, however, was a double-edged sword. While virtually all euthanasia advocates hailed it as a great victory, not everyone agreed it ought to be the last. One group within the euthanasia movement believed it should be the prelude to the legalization of both active euthanasia and physician-assisted suicide. Others, such as prominent physician (and ESA member) Walter Alvarez, even hoped that the acceptance of the living will would lead to a law permitting a physician "to end the useless days of a very dull idiot or a person who after a big stroke was left a human vegetable, unable to talk or to recognize his loved ones."[100] As long as success had eluded euthanasia activists, it was easy for disagreements over aims and strategy to be swept under the rug in the interests of collaborative attempts to win in the short run some measure of public support. With the first taste of success, conflicting expectations quickly surfaced, and the unity the movement had enjoyed for years rapidly dissolved in the 1970s.

V.

As the EEF drafted and distributed the living will and disseminated information on death and dying in the early 1970s, the first significant cracks in the euthanasia movement's ranks began to show. Individuals, dissatisfied that the EEF had temporarily forsaken efforts to lobby politicians for the legalization of euthanasia, decided to take matters into their own hands. One such activist was the Florida physician Walter Sackett, a Democratic state representative. Between 1968 and 1974, Sackett tried in vain to get the Florida legislature to pass bills enacting passive euthanasia and include "the right to die with dignity" in the state's bill of rights. Despite the interval of thirty years, his thinking was remarkably similar to that of early ESA president Foster Kennedy, who had argued that the people who really needed the right to die were not mentally competent and rational adults, but the mentally incompetent. Sackett's efforts earned him interviews on the Phil Donahue and Dick Cavett television shows and the CBS news program *60 Minutes*. They also made him a hero to those activists who had never given up the dream of achieving the legalization of euthanasia, but his campaign in the Sunshine State was soon mired in the kind of controversy that had plagued the movement in earlier decades.[101]

In common with other euthanasia advocates, Sackett had more than one motive for seeking euthanasia legislation. As a physician, he wanted immunity from prosecution if he were caught doing what he and many doctors were already doing. Polls in the 1960s showed that from 60 to 80 percent of American doctors let some of their patients die by withholding or withdrawing treatment.[102] In 1973 news broke that as many as forty-three deformed infants had been allowed to die with parental consent at the Yale-New Haven Hospital nursery, a reminder that Harry Haiselden's ideas were alive and well. The hospital's chief of staff said that allowing hopelessly ill patients to die "is accepted medical practice" and "nothing new."[103] As Sackett himself brazenly admitted in 1972, "I have let hundreds of people die."[104]

Sackett had been scarred by the death of his son in a 1960 automobile accident, and when he encountered situations where physicians were forced by law to keep brain-damaged children alive at all costs, he tended to imagine his son in the same circumstances. "If that were my child," he told the press in 1970, "I would hope he would be gone. If he got a cold, pneumonia, I would withhold antibiotics." But when Sackett added the state's potential "economic bankruptcy" as a reason for letting the mentally and physically handicapped die, he drew criticism. Had he not resorted to such inflammatory statements, it is conceivable that Florida would have passed the nation's first death with dignity law.[105]

Similar legislative initiatives coincided with Sackett's efforts in Florida. Thirty-five bills were introduced in twenty-two state legislatures between 1969 and 1976. While most were concerned with passive euthanasia, some (in Montana, Idaho, and Wisconsin) contained provisions for voluntary active euthanasia.[106] But besides Sackett, only one other state politician, Governor Tom McCall of Oregon, openly defended euthanasia legislation. Due to McCall's endorsement of the living will and passive euthanasia, the Oregon legislature introduced two euthanasia bills, but a public outcry and the militant opposition of Roman Catholic bishops forced Oregon euthanasia supporters to revise the bill to cover only passive euthanasia. By then the damage had been done, and in 1973 the Senate and House versions of the bill died in committee. Right-to-die activists in Oregon would have the last laugh, however. In 1997 Oregon became the first American state to legalize physician-assisted suicide.[107]

Other individuals had decided by the early 1970s to flout EEF policy and seek euthanasia legislation, foreshadowing the split that would develop in the movement in the late 1970s. The most notable dissident was Olive Ruth Russell, a Canadian-born educator and psychologist who, after her retirement from college teaching in 1962, dedicated the remainder of her life until her death in 1979 to the legalization of euthanasia. Russell's *Freedom to Die: Moral and Legal Aspects of Euthanasia* (1975), the first history of the euthanasia movement, was a milestone for the movement in itself, taking six years of exhaustive research and writing to complete. Besides anticipating the emergence in the 1980s of groups such as the Hemlock Society, which advocate active euthanasia, Russell was a throwback to the Progressivist spirit of the early ESA, in that she expressed strong support for the mercy killing of persons with disabilities without their consent. She also stood out as a formidable individual in whom many of the other driving forces behind the twentieth-century euthanasia movement intersected: Unitarianism, Humanism, and women's rights. Like most of her predecessors in the movement, she believed the struggle for the right to die was part of the ongoing effort to break "the stranglehold of tradition and religious dogma" and enact humane laws for a democratic society.[108] With one foot in the past and another in the future, Russell embodied the unresolved tension between paternalism and individual freedom that had marked the euthanasia movement virtually since its beginning.

Born in 1897, Russell, who held a Ph.D. in psychology, was heavily influenced by the educational theories of John Dewey, believing like him that psychology held the key to a vast reform of schooling, which, through its capacity to produce well-adjusted individuals, would strengthen democracy. Russell shared Dewey's faith that the right curricula could prepare students for the roles each was best suited to play in a society and economy that were growing increasingly complex. Like early ESA member Wyllistine Goodsell, whose influence she was exposed to while studying at Columbia University's Teachers' College in 1941, Russell subscribed to the Deweyite theory of social reconstructionism that called for schools to educate a new kind of citizen able to exercise his or her democratic responsibilities in the face of religious authoritarianism and the temptations of fascism. As with much of interwar educational progressivism, the theory of social reconstructionism was vague about where social planning ended and individual freedom began. It was similar to the notion, articulated by Humanists, Unitarians, and Ethical Culture theorists, that true freedom lay not in the pioneer individualism that had built

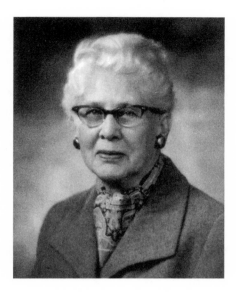

Olive Ruth Russell. *National Archives of Canada.*

the country but in creating a social environment that empowered individuals with the freedom to make choices that served noble ideals. This viewpoint later informed Russell's approach to euthanasia.

Russell too shared Goodsell's interest in women's rights, a trait nurtured in 1942 when she became the first woman psychologist in the Canadian army, and after World War II led the Canadian government's program to rehabilitate women veterans.[109] She emerged from her experience as a public servant with a firm belief that women should no longer suffer from sexual discrimination. Later in life, her commitment to women's rights led her to support birth control and abortion reform. Just as she defended the equality of women and approved of a woman's right to reproductive choice, so she approved of a person's right to choose the time, place, and manner of his or her death.[110]

Leaving the Canadian public service in 1947, Russell gradually became convinced of the righteousness of euthanasia on the basis of two poignant events in her life. Each experience left a distinct imprint on Russell's mind, and together they account for the seeming conflict between her support for individual freedom to choose death and her belief that the handicapped deserved a merciful death, whether or not they were able to choose.

Like so many others associated with the euthanasia movement, Russell was appalled by the spectacle of helpless and severely handicapped children who seemed to enjoy no quality of life. She and her college students made various visits to a nearby hospital. There they saw a hydrocephalic child "whose head was so heavy and his deformed body so tiny, he was helpless and bed-ridden, unable to talk, and doomed to lie there helplessly as long as his heart continued to beat." Russell decided that there was "something wrong with a society that requires a poor innocent child to lie there year after year in that helpless condition," and she vowed to change the laws so such individuals could be put out of their misery.[111]

Russell became a convert to euthanasia because she also witnessed her mother's painful death at the age of eighty-seven in 1955, another iconic experience for right-to-die advocates. Her mother endured rheumatoid arthritis for thirty-five years, the last twelve years of which were spent bed-ridden. Then her mother suffered a stroke that left her paralyzed and unable to eat solid food for three months; the last ten days of her life she could no longer take liquids. Despite her desire to die, conveyed to both her physician and daughter, there was nothing they could do legally, except make sure that no measures be taken to keep her alive. She eventually died of thirst and starvation. Reflecting on this grim spectacle, Russell concluded that God would have approved if her mother's physician had ended her suffering.[112]

These formative experiences, plus her dedication to ending injustice and human suffering, made Russell an impassioned defender of euthanasia, defining it as a merciful act administered by a physician to help a terminally ill patient who was trapped in "hopeless suffering or a meaningless existence." She rejected all eugenic rationales for euthanasia, and she condemned any program of state-imposed euthanasia. Instead, she stressed that voluntary active euthanasia should be legalized with the proper safeguards "to protect the rights of physicians and patients." A "right to die with dignity," to Russell, was a right all individuals within a free society should enjoy, including individuals who could not grant their informed consent. Rather than call this "involuntary" euthanasia, she preferred "non-voluntary." Her version of "non-voluntary" euthanasia had to be requested by the patients' parents or guardians.[113]

Armed with these ideas, in the 1960s Russell and her longtime companion Ruth Roettinger went seeking the "dynamic leadership" of the euthanasia cause they hoped for, but they learned to their disappointment that the EEF merely supported the right to refuse treatment. Never one to keep her opinions to herself, Russell criticized EEF policy throughout the 1970s for being too cautious.[114]

In the meantime, she resolved to keep the memory of "the early pioneers" of the ESA alive and decided, on Joseph Fletcher's advice, to write *Freedom to Die*. This book depicted the rise of the right-to-die movement as a triumphal story of steady progress leading to the late twentieth century.[115] All that impeded this march of progress, she wrote, were the self-interest and ignorance of reactionary groups—chiefly organized medicine and religion. But Russell's eagerness to describe religion and medicine as obstacles to reason, democracy, and humanity meant she sidestepped controversial chapters of the movement's past while misrepresenting others. She paid virtually no attention to the many eugenic supporters of euthanasia in the ESA's early years. On the most serious question—the link between Nazism and euthanasia—Russell dismissed Leo Alexander's "slippery slope" thesis that the murderous policies of the Third Reich started with "small beginnings" predating Hitler's rise to power. Russell drew firm distinctions between "the cold-blooded, secretive, and deceptive program of the Nazis" and the open and heavily safeguarded methods she advocated. As she argued, if there was a danger of a lapse into Nazism, it lay in accepting "the idea that secret agents of the state—doctors or others—should be permitted or ordered to terminate the lives of those they decide were unwanted or 'useless eaters.' " The danger, she maintained, did *not* lie in "the belief that life sometimes becomes not worth living," a belief she shared with many in the euthanasia movement.[116] In other words, she was supremely confident that nothing like what had happened in the Third Reich could ever happen in America.

Because Russell never lived to see her dreams fulfilled, one can only speculate whether she was sincere in her rejection of state euthanasia programs. Her less than discriminate admiration for people such as Walter Sackett, whose own views raised eyebrows in other quarters, was not only characteristic of many euthanasia supporters but also casts doubts on her bona fides. She was similar to many defenders of the right to die in that her eagerness to achieve the legalization of euthanasia probably influenced her to hold back her more paternalistic views until the day voluntary active euthanasia was legalized. As an activist, she believed tactical considerations dictated that she keep her private convictions quiet for the time being.

Russell's readiness to act independently of the ESA drew her to the American Humanist Association (AHA), the descendant of Potter's First Humanist Society and, even earlier, Robert Ingersoll's and Felix Adler's ideas. The AHA, which bestowed a Humanist Pioneer Award on Russell in 1977, had been founded in 1941 and over the course of its history has had firm ties to the Ethical Culture movement. In fact, Humanism, the notion that all old beliefs should be shed and replaced by a faith in human nature and intelligence, has been defined as the common philosophy of both the AHA and Ethical Culture.[117] While the Ethical Culture societies had not taken an official stand on euthanasia by the 1970s, the AHA, as early as 1959, had urged its membership to "work for changes in existing laws" to permit voluntary active euthanasia,[118] and many prominent members of both groups have done so since.[119] Their journals, *The Humanist* and *The Ethical Outlook*, have also published numerous articles on euthanasia, virtually all supportive. In 1973, the AHA recognized "an individual's right to die with dignity, euthanasia, and the right to suicide" as fundamental civil liberties. The next year, "A Plea for Beneficent Euthanasia" was published in *The Humanist*, an "appeal to an enlightened public opinion to transcend traditional taboos" and support the legalization of both passive and active euthanasia. It was signed by (among others) Russell, Joseph Fletcher, biologist Linus Pauling, philosopher Sidney Hook, and AHA president Betty Chambers. One of the AHA's programs was the National Commission for Beneficent Euthanasia (NCBE), an organization formed in 1974 and advocating both active and passive euthanasia, with Russell serving in an advisory capacity.[120] Humanists tended to support the right to die because they "consider themselves open-minded," an AHA document read,

> . . . free from illogical or unproved dogmatic assumptions. Our customs and laws seem based on either the premise that death is the most terrible thing that can happen, regardless of circumstances, or the premise that our lives belong to a deity who demands every effort to postpone death. Some of us cannot accept either. The latter, being a religious concept, has no place in the laws of a country having constitutional separation

of church and state. Humanists do not place the responsibility for suffering upon a deity, but accept personal responsibility to correct the evils of our society. We value individual freedom, human rights.[121]

The "Plea" denied there was any distinction between active and passive euthanasia. It maintained that if society accepted the withdrawal of life-prolonging techniques in terminal illness, then there was no logical or ethical reason not to accept "the administration of increasing doses of drugs (such as morphine) to relieve suffering, until the dosage, of necessity, reaches the lethal stage." This, of course, was the Catholic "double-effect" theory.[122]

One signatory to the "Plea" whose life and career epitomized the congruence of Humanism, Ethical Culture, and euthanasia was Algernon Black. Born in 1900 to Russian Jewish immigrants, Black at an early age won a scholarship to the Ethical Culture School in New York City. When Felix Adler died in 1933, Black was instrumental in helping to transform Ethical Culture's message into support for social programs to meet the crises of the Depression. Black went on to advocate racial desegregation, civil rights, and nuclear disarmament, and he also joined the ESA and the Association for Voluntary Sterilization in the 1950s, undeterred by these organizations' eugenic pasts. In 1963, he emphasized that euthanasia, because it "originates in man's concern for his fellowman and his compassion for one who is suffering unbearably," was an ideal cause for the Ethical Culture movement to support. "If we had a more ethical world," Black contended, "we would be able to help one another live, and we would be able to help one another to die."[123]

As for Russell, her admiration for Unitarianism, like her connection to Humanism, was another bridge between the ESA's past and the euthanasia movement's future. In 1988, the Unitarian Universalist Association passed a national resolution affirming the right to die, becoming the first religious body in America to do so.[124] This was the culmination of a long history of close relations between Unitarians and the euthanasia movements on both sides of the Atlantic Ocean, harking back to the 1930s. Russell, although she never joined a Unitarian congregation, had concluded by the 1960s that much of the theology imparted to her by her Methodist parents was superstitious nonsense, and Unitarianism, with its advocacy of the social gospel, its opposition to fatalism, its rejection of specific creeds, and its encouragement to individuals to create their own value systems, was a breath of fresh air to her. To Russell, there was an obvious harmony between Unitarianism and belief in the right to die.[125]

Russell's interest in euthanasia intensified in the last years of her life as her own health faltered badly. In this respect, too, she personified many of the concerns of health care consumers, especially women. As she told advice columnist Ann Landers in 1977, for fifteen years she had consulted five different doctors about the acute pain she felt in her head, what would later be diagnosed as Paget's Disease, a chronic illness caused by the weakening, enlarging, and deformation of the bones. This experience confirmed her suspicions that too many male doctors were willing to dismiss the symptoms of women patients as hysterical, a key complaint of the women's movement about the medical profession. When she was hospitalized in 1975, she found herself "hooked up" to an oxygen machine and monitor. She decided at that moment that if her life became "meaningless," she would ask a doctor to end her life, which her personal physician did on 25 May 1979, after her kidneys failed and she lapsed into a coma.[126]

Russell's support of euthanasia was also tied to her interests in the population control movement. She advocated euthanasia as one method for dealing with the "surging rise in the number of physically and mentally crippled children" caused by the "population explosion."[127] Nor was she alone in linking euthanasia and population control. Population controllers William Vogt, author of the bestseller *Road to Survival* (1948), and P. K. Whelpton, one-time director of the Scripps Foundation for Research in Population Problems, were ESA members.[128]

The best example of the overlap between the euthanasia and population control movements was the millionaire Hugh Moore (1887–1972), who, when he died in 1972, left the EEF over $1,000,000, one-quarter of his residuary estate.[129] Opinionated and abrasive, Moore used his immense wealth, thanks to his invention of the Dixie Cup, the first sanitary paper drinking vessel, to warn about the dangers of the earth's dramatic population growth in the modern era, what he called the "population bomb." (In fact Moore coined the phrase the "population bomb" before Stanford University biologist Paul Ehrlich made it famous in 1968.) Moore blamed communism's inroads into the developing world on the poverty, scarcity, and misery created by population growth. By 1961, he had raised hundreds of thousands of dollars for the cause of reducing population levels.[130] In later years, he also threw his support behind environmentalism, abortion rights, and euthanasia.[131] A longtime foe of Catholicism's condemnation of artificial contraception and population control, he helped to organize a massive counterattack against Pope Paul VI's *Humanae Vitae* (1968), which reaffirmed Church teaching against birth control and sterilization.[132]

Having concluded that sterilization was the best contraceptive method of population control, Moore capitalized on the Human Betterment Association of America's desperate need for funding to co-opt HBAA policy in the 1960s and reshape it to suit his own agenda. Under Moore, the HBAA became the Association for Voluntary Sterilization and shifted its focus from the domestic scene to overseas, from widening access to sterilization services in the United States to introducing mass sterilization programs in overpopulated and underdeveloped countries, such as India.[133]

Eugenic notions were never far from the core of Moore's thinking about population control. In 1966, he cited predictions that America's population would exceed 350,000,000 in the next thirty years, resulting in "over-crowded cities, polluted air and water, countless unwanted and suffering children, skyrocketing taxes for welfare! Half of the babies now born in some cities are from indigent families on relief. Need we say more?"[134] Officially, Moore supported only voluntary sterilization, but like other activists in the population control field he believed that, unless elective sterilization was widespread, especially among those classes and in those countries that most needed it, then broad programs of compulsory sterilization would be urgently required. Moore's views and actions, seemingly targeting vulnerable and disadvantaged social groups, rekindled bad memories of the coercive eugenic sterilization practices of America's past. His attitude might be best summed up as: "voluntary sterilization now, or else."[135]

As the 1960s unfolded, Moore befriended Paul Ehrlich, author of the best-seller *The Population Bomb* (1968), and supported pro-abortion organizations such as the National Association for the Repeal of Abortion Laws (NARAL).[136] Moore did not defend abortion and birth control because he thought women deserved these individual rights, but because he wanted to use them to reduce population around the globe. His endorsement of abortion and birth con-

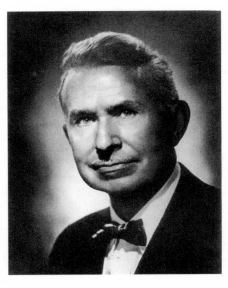

Hugh Moore. *Seeley G. Mudd Manuscript Library, Princeton University.*

trol was a sign that his overall message blended with the shifting cultural mood of the country, one that teetered uneasily between authoritarianism and individual freedom.

Thus, by the time he began his involvement in the euthanasia movement in the late 1960s, Moore had cultivated a hodgepodge of interests in population control, environmentalism, and abortion reform as well as a poorly concealed sympathy for coercive public policy. He and his wife, Louise Wilde Moore, started contributing financially to the ESA in the mid-1960s, and attended the first EEF meeting in 1968.[137] The generosity of his 1972 $1,000,000 gift was astounding, in view of the EEF's modest size and the fact that Moore had given few indications that he was deeply concerned about euthanasia. Undoubtedly, his late-blooming interest in euthanasia was due to a growing preoccupation with his own mortality, but philosophically it also made sense given his other interests in life.[138] After his death, Moore's memory would be kept alive by his wife, Louise, who remained active in the movement into the 1990s.

Moore was not the only wealthy benefactor of euthanasia in the 1970s who was vitally interested in abortion and population control. John D. Rockefeller 3rd, Moore's compatriot in the population control movement, was showing similar signs of shifting his attention to euthanasia just before his untimely death in 1978. Rockefeller's views on population control were never as heavy-handed as Moore's, and by promoting gay rights and sex education in the 1970s he was endorsing causes that sharply conflicted with Moore's more conservative opinions. But their attitudes toward euthanasia were remarkably similar. Rockefeller gave Concern for Dying (CFD) $14,500 to help stage a conference entitled "Death, Dying, and Decision-Making," held in San Francisco, 16–18 November 1978. Within the euthanasia movement there were expectations that Rockefeller was preparing to do even more for the cause, before a car accident in Tarrytown, New York, cut short his life. In May 1976 Rockefeller had met with officials from both CFD and the Society for the Right to Die and expressed his particular interest in "active euthanasia" for the terminally ill and severely disabled infants. This led euthanasia advocates to hope that Rockefeller would agree to chair a broad-based committee to investigate the right to die. Rockefeller's private thoughts on euthanasia died with him, but had he not died when he did there would have been nothing surprising, given the trends of the day and the historical trajectory of his interests, if eventually he had become a preeminent leader of the movement.[139]

At first sight, the sympathy felt by population controllers Moore and Rockefeller might suggest that they looked to euthanasia as an actual means of curbing population growth. With the escalating fears about Malthusian scenarios, fanned in no small measure by doomsayers such as Moore, activists (including Ruth Russell) did cite the specter of an overcrowded, polluted planet as a reason for choosing euthanasia.

Some euthanasia advocates acted on these beliefs. Henry Van Dusen, former president of the Union Theological Seminary and original signatory of the 1948 ESA clergymen's statement on euthanasia, committed suicide with his wife in 1975. Both were in failing health, he disabled from a stroke and she suffering from worsening arthritis. They ended their lives because they saw no dignity in living any longer under increasing medical care, but they also thought that in a world of growing population, declining space, and too many mouths to feed, they were consuming valuable resources. The Van Dusens agreed that it was a misuse of medical science to keep terminally ill people alive simply because the technology was available.[140]

The interest of population controllers in the right to die is another example of how the euthanasia movement dovetailed with contemporaneous fashionable crusades throughout the twentieth century, a trend that stretched back to the heyday of social Darwinism and eugenics. But this was not simply a case of intellectual fashion, of activists jumping on bandwagons in an effort to gain credibility. There was a certain philosophic symmetry uniting eugenics, euthanasia, population control, birth control, and abortion reform. Practically, there were obvious links among them, such as the use of euthanasia as both a eugenic and population control method. But more importantly, what tied these various causes together was a common belief among their supporters that they were breaking what Russell called "the stranglehold of tradition and religious dogma," the barriers that allegedly prevented individual human beings from realizing their freedom.[141] This emancipationist agenda, while borrowing from the cultural mood of the 1970s, also recalled elements of Progressivism and the social reconstructionist theories of the 1930s that Russell and others had been weaned on, as well as the rhetoric surrounding the birth control campaign and the anti-Catholicism that had punctuated much of the struggle in the late 1940s over the separation of church and state. In Russell's words, now that "freedom of choice regarding planned parenthood, abortion, and birth control has been won," euthanasia was "the next great freedom."[142] But at the heart of Russell's liberationist agenda was the same fundamental ambiguity about the boundaries between voluntarism and involuntarism, a right to privacy and the right of the community to defend itself, that had dogged earlier generations of euthanasia proponents. Thus, while things had changed a great deal for the euthanasia movement by the 1970s, in other respects they had not changed much at all.

VI.

The actions and words of individuals such as Russell and Moore indicated there was a group that, as the 1970s wore on, was growing restless with what it thought was the euthanasia movement's overly cautious direction. This group, headed by Joseph Fletcher, revived the old ESA in 1974 and renamed it the Society for the Right to Die (SRD). The founding of the SRD marked a renewed dedication to pursuing the legalization of active euthanasia, a reenergized campaign to seek euthanasia laws through the political process. But just as this was happening, another group within the movement, and clustered within the ranks of the EEF/EEC, was arriving at the very different conclusion that legislative reform beyond the recognition of living wills was unnecessary. In 1978, this group changed the name of the EEC to Concern for Dying (CFD), a signal that its focus was shifting from giving people the constitutional freedom to die to other issues, such as hospice and palliative care and better communications among patients, their families, and health care providers. This difference of opinion would harden into a bitter, gut-wrenching battle in 1979–80 that tore the movement apart and resulted in the official separation of CFD and SRD. Out of the wrangling emerged not two but three different American right-to-die organizations, each with its own agenda and charismatic leadership. In the 1980s, for the first time an international euthanasia movement also crystallized, as right-to-die advocacy suddenly ceased to be limited to the United States and Great Britain. Sensationalist media coverage of the Karen Ann Quinlan and Nancy Cruzan tragedies would help to personalize the already highly emotional issue of death with dignity. Simultaneously, American euthanasia activists would face their most formidable opposition since the 1940s in the form of the pro-life movement, once again closely identified with the Catholic Church, but in the 1980s strengthened by the support of countless Protestant evangelicals.

Thus, as the 1980s dawned, a new chapter was opening in the history of the euthanasia movement in twentieth-century America. More Americans than ever believed in a right to die, but agreement about what the right to die actually meant was increasingly difficult to reach. At the same time, the movement's unity had been shattered and battle lines (both old and new) had been drawn. To some long-time members of the movement, this was tragic. To others, more optimistically, it was an opportunity for reorganization, remobilization, and reinvention. But the bottom line was that such divisiveness severely compromised the chances of the movement to win American public opinion precisely when attitudes seemed more receptive than ever. The fallout from this state of affairs would begin to show as the end of the twentieth century approached.

5

Not That Simple, 1975–1990

When American euthanasia advocates gathered in New York City in 1974, the mood should have been euphoric. Over the previous decade, the progress of the movement had been astonishing. Speaking openly about death and dying had become fashionable, and a majority of Americans (53 percent) believed that doctors should be allowed to end the lives of terminally ill patients by painless methods if the patients and their families requested it. An even larger majority (62 percent) supported the right of terminally ill patients to refuse unwanted medical treatment.[1] Internationally, other countries were in the process of forming their own euthanasia organizations. It seemed as if interest in the right to die was sweeping the whole world.

However, the overall mood among euthanasia proponents in 1974 was far from buoyant. The Euthanasia Society of America had just been reactivated and renamed the Society for the Right to Die (SRD), the opening act in a sectarian drama that would shortly grip a movement whose unity had long been taken for granted. A split was beginning to form, between those who felt better end-of-life care and more discussion about death with dignity were the top priorities, and those who wanted to transform the growing popular acceptance of the right to refuse unwanted treatment into the decriminalization of active euthanasia and medically assisted suicide. This divergence of opinion would ultimately cause a bitter turf war within the euthanasia movement and slow its progress as the century drew to a close.[2]

These wrangles were simply a reflection of the broader developments in the national debate over the right to die in the 1970s and 1980s. The heartrending plight of Karen Ann Quinlan, the founding of Derek Humphry's Hemlock Society, the formation of the World Federation of Right-to-Die Societies, and the stunning AIDS epidemic radicalized many euthanasia advocates in the 1970s and 1980s. In the ensuing controversy, some Americans concluded that the questions surrounding euthanasia were growing larger, not smaller, but others believed that the right to die was as clear-cut as it had always been and sought to return the movement to its historic roots during the early years of the Euthanasia Society of America. The efforts of these latter activists testified to their deep conviction that the time had finally come in America to legalize active euthanasia.

I.

By the mid-1970s, few within the American euthanasia movement were more uneasy about where it was headed than Donald McKinney. In his first years with the EEF, McKinney had shared the enthusiasm of others in the organization as donations flowed in and membership rolls grew. As he recalled in 1976: "Years ago, when we were so eager to break the barrier of silence surrounding euthanasia, and some of us would willingly sit up all night to be able to get on talk shows, and would accept any invitations to talk with students and other groups, the questions of euthanasia seemed much simpler, and the goals far clearer than they do today."[3] Back then, McKinney believed that the issues raised by euthanasia were "as critical to our time as were those of family planning a generation or so ago."[4] He readily subscribed to Joseph Fletcher's dictum that "death control, like birth control, is a matter of human dignity—without it we are puppets."[5]

But by the mid-1970s, McKinney was no longer convinced Fletcher

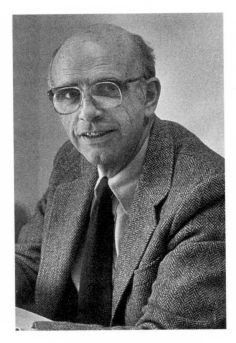

Donald W. McKinney. *First Unitarian Church, Brooklyn, N.Y.*

was right. He had come to doubt Fletcher's theory that active and passive euthanasia were essentially the same thing.[6] He found himself agreeing with a growing belief among bioethicists that "those treasured goals of 'death with dignity,' 'right to die,' etc., are more clichés than clear and compelling goals." By 1976, he had decided that euthanasia and birth control had little in common. Defying a tradition within the euthanasia movement that dated back to the days of William Robinson, Charles Potter, Margaret Sanger, Eleanor Dwight Jones, and Robert Latou Dickinson, and bucking the trend that had seen many Unitarians become stalwart defenders of active euthanasia, McKinney argued that death control was "a far more awesome matter than birth control."[7] Reproductive choice, which he supported, was not the same thing as personal choice in dying.

McKinney's conclusion that euthanasia and family planning were two very different matters marked the beginnings of a new current within the euthanasia movement, one that put him on a collision course with Joseph Fletcher and some of the SRD's board. The SRD, led by people such as Fletcher, tax lawyer Sidney Rosoff, psychiatrist

Florence Clothier, and longtime ESA member Ruth Proskauer Smith, spent much of the 1970s working with their allies in various states to obtain living will legislation. The SRD never campaigned for active euthanasia, and some members were highly uneasy about the practice (especially "Dear Abby" Van Buren). But the long-term goal of other, key SRD members was legalizing the actual hastening of a patient's death through a doctor's intervention. Fletcher, Rosoff, Clothier, Smith, and others tended to see the legislative recognition of living wills not as their ultimate goal but as a prelude to an equally concerted effort to lobby politicians for the enactment of active euthanasia laws, and (in Clothier's case at least) an even wider expansion of euthanasia to include deformed infants and severely handicapped adults.[8]

In this campaign to legalize active euthanasia Fletcher stood front and center. As he declared in 1973, "soft-pedaling the euthanasia question in favor of the when-to-let-them-die question" was "old-hat already."[9] "The plain fact" was that

[e]very day in a hundred hospitals across the land decisions are made clinically that the line has been crossed from prolonging genuinely human life to only prolonging subhuman dying, and when that judgment is made respirators are turned off, life-perpetuating intravenous infusions stopped, proposed surgery canceled, and drugs countermanded. So-called "Code 90" stickers are put on many record-jackets, indicating "Give no intensive care or resuscitation."[10]

To Fletcher, "soft-pedaling" euthanasia once had been useful, but it was time for Americans to consider going farther and legalizing both active voluntary euthanasia and active involuntary euthanasia. In 1974 he stated that if the euthanasia movement "wants to give some kind of leadership and activity along the front, I think we'd better get back to what the [ESA] was talking about when it came into being, and continued to talk about until ten years ago." Therein lay a significant difference between Fletcher and McKinney: Fletcher thought the country was finally catching up to what the old ESA had preached for years, while McKinney believed it was the euthanasia movement that had to catch up to the country's rapidly shifting views on death and dying.[11]

These differences of opinion between Fletcher and McKinney

were played out on the larger, organizational level. Virtually from the moment the ESA was reactivated in 1974 as the SRD, it and the EEC went their separate ways. Even the choice of Society for the Right to Die as the name for the old ESA reflected the divergence of purpose between the two. The SRD board rejected the word euthanasia because, as "Dear Abby" stated in 1974, "a bill with the word 'euthanasia' in it will never get passed."[12] The SRD board also dropped euthanasia because it wanted to distinguish itself from the more moderate and cautious EEC.[13]

For public consumption, however, the two organizations remained allied until 1980. They shared the same office in Manhattan. In 1978 it was agreed that the SRD would stop soliciting its own funds and let the nonprofit CFD grant it operating funds from donations to both groups, but some EEC members worried that it was merely a "front" for the SRD.[14] Shortly after the 1978 funding decision, SRD representatives were told that "the affiliate relationship" between the two groups would be "dissolved."[15] CFD promised it would continue to fund the SRD, but later in 1979 the promise virtually evaporated when CFD announced it would fund the SRD only for another year at a paltry $4,900 a month. The SRD's staff were also told to vacate their office space.[16]

The reasons for these events lay in the fact that, philosophically, CFD and the SRD had diverged dramatically during the 1970s. The SRD was an "activist" organization, CFD president Kay Mali stated in September 1979, but "Concern's [aim] is one of philosophic exploration of issues and their ramifications, based on the belief that the best form of teaching is to present all sides of a problem. There are, moreover, [CFD] members who have serious reservations as to the wisdom of the legislative approach in general." The subtext to her remarks was the growing discontent among many CFD members about the comments in favor of active euthanasia uttered by individuals such as Fletcher. If CFD was to provide funding for the SRD, yet not exercise any influence over the latter's policy, then to Mali it was best for both groups to separate.[17]

Exerting influence over SRD policy was an important issue, given the pronounced views in favor of active euthanasia of people such as Fletcher and Florence Clothier. Clothier, born in 1903 in Wynnewood, Pennsylvania, was in many respects a throwback to the thinking that inspired the ESA in the days of Charles Potter. Indeed, she remembered hearing Potter speak on the topic of euthanasia in

Boston "in about 1939." "Every 'kook' in Boston went," she remi-
nisced. "Tomatoes were not actually thrown at the clergyman, but
[Potter] was bombasted verbally. It was a nearly violent
performance."[18]

Following a well-trod path, Clothier came to the euthanasia movement after leadership roles in the birth control movement. Her husband had died in 1956 after suffering a "painful protracted terminal
illness with cancer," an important reason behind her interest in euthanasia.[19] But having joined the movement, she, like so many other
defenders of euthanasia, contended that there was a fundamental
kinship uniting "the issues of family planning, birth control, abortions and euthanasia." "Some of these things concern the beginning
of life and some the end, but they all concern the *quality* of life."[20]
What prevented society from accepting these practices, she argued,
was the "Judeo-Christian obsession with prolonged existence."[21]

Clothier, unlike Joseph Fletcher, did not try to hide her support
of involuntary euthanasia. She conceded that the 1970s were too
soon to advocate voluntary active euthanasia, but she endorsed both
it and the "compassionate involuntary" euthanasia of "accidents of
nature." Echoing Sackett and Russell, Clothier stated that "[h]aving
spent time on the back wards of state hospitals and schools for the
retarded," she was in favor of physicians "actively terminat[ing] the
life of an infant with no hope of anything except a vegetative institutional existence." For these cases, she thought it unadvisable to
even consult with parents. "Far better for [the parents] to believe
that their hopelessly defective handicapped baby was born dead or
died soon after birth." For the "less flagrant 'accidents of nature,' "
such as "mongoloid babies, severe cerebral palsy, extreme physical
deformities, etc.," parents "should be appraised in so far as possible
of the long-term prognosis and should be helped to reach a humane
and wise decision in terms of the best interests of their baby and
their family."[22]

However, Clothier (like Sackett) also lamented the "emotional
and physical drain" on health care personnel who took care of such
people, in addition to the consumption of valuable resources that
could be used to help "those less handicapped." In a sentiment that
was shared by more than a few within the movement, Clothier argued that in the short term activists should advocate only voluntary
passive euthanasia. But "when that becomes legal and generally accepted," she declared in 1977, it was time to "begin a public edu-

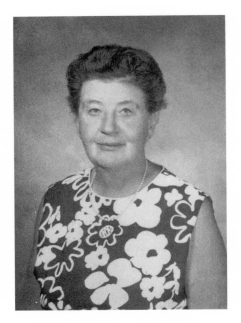

Florence Clothier. *Schlesinger Library, Radcliffe Institute, Harvard University.*

cational program" recommending active voluntary and involuntary euthanasia.[23]

Clothier's outspoken defense of euthanasia for the handicapped underlined the philosophic differences between the CFD's board and individuals like her. "A clash of personalities," primarily involving Sidney Rosoff and Ruth Proskauer Smith, made these differences even more divisive.[24] Rosoff's and Smith's names kept coming up as sources of friction in the terse exchanges between the two organizations in 1979. Rosoff, born in 1924, became an ESA member in 1961 and assisted Pauline Taylor in her efforts to attain tax-exempt status for the organization. In the 1970s Rosoff served on the boards of CFD and the SRD, but he gradually fell out with CFD board members over the issue of seeking right-to-die legislation. Although he and the SRD board restricted their energies to winning living will legislation in the 1970s, his activities as president of the World Federation of Right-to-Die Societies and of Derek Humphry's Hemlock Society indicate that he supported the old ESA strategy of first securing the legalization of passive euthanasia as a way of preparing public opinion to accept active euthanasia later.[25]

The perception that Rosoff was difficult to get along with also applied to his SRD colleague and friend Ruth Proskauer Smith.[26] Over the last half of the twentieth century, few Americans did more than the feisty Smith to increase public awareness of euthanasia, family planning, and abortion. Still alert and as dedicated as ever to the right to die when interviewed in 2000, Smith was born in 1907 in Deal, New Jersey, and educated at Manhattan's Ethical Culture school, another example of the enduring ties between Ethical Culture and the struggle for legalized euthanasia. Although her father was an Al Smith Democrat, she soon gravitated toward the anti-Catholicism of Paul Blanshard, Eleanor Dwight Jones, and Protestants and Other Americans United for Separation of Church and State.[27] When Catholics opposed the ESA, Smith tended to view the issue of euthanasia in the same terms as she did birth control and government funding for parochial schools. To her mind, the Church was trying to impose its values on individual Americans, breaching the walls dividing church and state.

When she joined the ESA in 1954, Ruth Smith already knew about the organization through her mother, a board member who often hosted ESA meetings in her Manhattan apartment. Earlier, Smith had been a birth control activist in Massachusetts, and from 1954 to 1956 served as an administrator at gynecologist Alan Guttmacher's contraceptive clinic at the Mount Sinai Hospital in New York City. Leaving the clinic one day to attend a meeting of the ESA at her mother's apartment, she was pleasantly surprised to find Guttmacher catching a bus for the same destination.[28]

At roughly the same time, Ruth Smith met Joseph Fletcher, whose son was dating her daughter, and she convinced Fletcher to become more involved in the ESA. The Fletcher-Smith-Guttmacher connection grew even firmer when, in 1955, she became executive director of the Human Betterment Association of America (HBAA), on whose board both men agreed to serve, a move that strengthened the ties between that organization and the ESA.[29]

Her mother's death in 1957 turned her into a euthanasia activist. Despite the fact that Alice Naumburg Proskauer had written a letter before her terminal illness, specifying how she wanted to be allowed to die, her wishes were ignored by her physician, and she suffered greatly before dying. Smith was just one of many euthanasia advocates who were deeply pained by witnessing the protracted death of a friend or relative, but she was also the sort of euthanasia proponent whose personal brushes with the deaths of loved ones were made more philosophically meaningful by her overall approach to matters of sex, fertility, reproduction, and death. For someone who already believed in the right to personal autonomy in birth control, the spectacle of another person's dying wishes being ignored was as egregious an injustice as a woman being forced to bear children she did not want. In Smith's own words, her interests in abortion, birth control, and euthanasia were "all of a piece."[30]

In the 1960s, Smith campaigned for the reform of abortion laws, but as time wore on, she devoted more and more of her energies to euthanasia. She was responsible for Luis Kutner broaching the idea of the living will at an ESA meeting in 1967, and thanks to her involvement in the HBAA, she talked Hugh Moore into donating some of his wealth to the EEF. By the time of the 1980 CFD/SRD split, she, like Rosoff, was a formidable member of both boards.[31]

However, if Smith's powers of persuasion worked with Fletcher, Guttmacher, Kutner, and Moore, they proved to be less effective with CFD members who complained that both Smith and Rosoff "represent[ed] a personality problem." Smith admitted she kept "needling Concern to make up its mind on [its] program. They apparently are getting tired of my asking." That she was pressuring them none too subtly to adopt a stance favorable to active euthanasia made her behavior all the more annoying to CFD members.[32]

Money matters proved to be just as divisive as the differences over philosophy and personalities. By 1978 CFD was running a deficit of almost $80,000. The distribution of living wills, once a cash cow for the group, was bringing in less and less money. The growing suspicion that the SRD's legislative program would switch to promotion of active euthanasia, and thus scare off potential benefactors, was also a worry for CFD. Collaboration with the SRD led to allegations that CFD was "really a cover-up, really an active euthanasia organization in disguise."[33] CFD's board took all these factors into consideration and decided it was time for the two organizations to part ways. The unity of the American euthanasia movement had come to end.[34]

Once matters reached the separation stage, pretense of amicability quickly vanished, and bickering broke out over Hugh Moore's $1 million bequest.[35] The SRD filed a lawsuit against CFD in late 1979 demanding all funds, including the Hugh Moore bequest, that CFD had raised to support the quest for euthanasia legislation.[36] In the lawsuit, settled out of court in 1985, CFD agreed to provide a grant of $275,000 to the SRD (by then a nonprofit corporation).³⁷ Most members of the two organizations probably knew nothing about the bad feelings generated by the split, but to the boards of both groups the lawsuit had been gut-wrenching. To Fletcher, the whole business reminded him of "patricide." Rosoff compared CFD's actions with those of a "child [who] is ashamed of the parent and wants to sever relations." He found the proposal of separation "destructive for the movement."³⁸ These bitter emotions would fester for the next ten years until events threw both organizations back together again, another sign of the shifting agendas motivating people in the euthanasia movement in the seventies and eighties.

What was obvious during the CFD/SRD split was that the entire euthanasia movement was in flux.³⁹ Most agreed that important decisions had to be made about the movement's future course, but agreement on what decisions ought to be made proved to be elusive. What were the movement's ultimate goals? After living wills, what? Were they the answer? What about assisted suicide and active euthanasia? The actions of individuals such as Donald McKinney reflected a mounting caution about the ESA's traditional goal of state laws permitting individuals to petition their physicians to assist them in dying while conferring immunity from prosecution on their doctors who agreed to help. CFD members felt that legislation "brings in government," when the whole matter of death with dignity was "better left to the individual."⁴⁰ For its part, the SRD's board continued to limit its support to the enactment of living will legislation; but suspicions that many on the SRD's board were really interested in assisted suicide and active euthanasia were generally accurate and would be borne out by events in the 1980s.

II.

As tensions between the two Manhattan-based euthanasia groups mounted, a somber series of events was unfolding, involving the fate of a pretty twenty-one-year-old named Karen Ann Quinlan. On 14 April 1974 Quinlan fell into an irreversible coma at a party in suburban New Jersey, possibly because she had been mixing alcohol and the tranquilizer Valium. Taken to hospital, she was hooked up to a respirator and tubes providing her with hydration and nutrition. When she persisted in her vegetative state for months, her parents went to court to have her taken off the respirator. They eventually succeeded in March 1976, but Karen Ann Quinlan, even after being detached from the respirator, lived for another nine years until she died of pneumonia in 1985.

As poignant as Quinlan's personal fate was, it was overshadowed by the public controversy over her right to die, recalling other moments in the nation's history when euthanasia had similarly captivated American public interest, such as the Bollinger baby death, Charlotte Perkins Gilman's suicide, and Hermann Sander's trial. But no prior episode in the history of euthanasia in America had garnered so much media attention nationally and internationally. Quinlan became an instant (if unlikely) celebrity, as her high school yearbook photograph was flashed across television screens and the front pages of newspapers around the world.[41] Her misfortune drove home the lesson that, in the modern age of new medical technology and attitudes toward death and dying, euthanasia had evolved into an exceedingly complex issue. This dawning realization humbled some individuals such as Donald McKinney, but others attempted to capitalize on the ambiguities surrounding the Quinlan case and argue that there were no legal, philosophic, or ethical barriers to making a right to die a constitutional freedom that all Americans ought to enjoy.

At first glance, the ruling of the New Jersey Supreme Court on 31 March 1976 that Karen Ann Quinlan could be detached from her respirator was a victory for her Roman Catholic parents. They had argued that the life-sustaining treatment their daughter had received constituted "extraordinary" treatment and, in the spirit of Pope Pius XII, could be discontinued. But while the court had agreed with the Quinlans' wishes, its decision was much less a victory for Catholic biomedical ethics than it was a groundbreaking, legal first step for right-to-die advocates. The Quinlan decision followed the 1965 *Griswold v. Connecticut* and 1973 *Roe v. Wade* U.S. Supreme Court rulings that Americans enjoyed a constitutional right to privacy, and stated that this right can be exercised when a terminally ill patient wishes to withhold or withdraw life support. Thus, the Quinlans benefitted from prior judicial rulings that had decriminalized contraception and abortion, two practices the Quinlans' church prohibited. But the Quinlan decision also stated that "Karen's right to privacy may be asserted on her behalf by her guardian under the peculiar circumstances here present." The "peculiar circumstances" included the significant fact that Karen had never signed a living will nor made her end-of-life wishes known clearly. As Princeton University medical ethicist Paul Ramsey argued, *In re Quinlan* went "a long way toward obliterating the distinction between voluntary and involuntary euthanasia and weakening legal protection of life from involuntary euthanasia." Yale Kamisar, speaking at a National Right to Life convention in Boston in 1976, concurred that the New Jersey Supreme Court might have "provided the euthanasiasts with something that has eluded them for decades—the bridge between voluntary and involuntary euthanasia."[42]

Thus, "*In re Quinlan* was the *Brown v. Board of Education* of the right-to-die movement."[43] Some in the movement took the ruling as a legal signal to begin open support of active euthanasia in the form of physician-assisted suicide.[44] To the emerging pro-life movement, however, the decision was a travesty of justice, a blow to the doctrine of the sanctity of life, and its members mobilized at the state level to combat the legalization of living wills.

A strong and dedicated movement in America seeking to roll back *Roe v. Wade* and defeat the forces of euthanasia slowly but steadily gathered strength in the 1970s. Initially, Catholics led the pro-life crusade, whose first victory occurred in 1976 when Congress placed restrictions on federal funding of abortions. Antiabortion groups formed an umbrella organization, the National Right to Life Committee, which by the late 1970s wielded a $1.3 million budget. A New Right began materializing, supported by conservative activists and a renewed Protestant fundamentalism under the leadership of evangelicals, including Moral Majority preacher Jerry Falwell. Then, in 1980, the pro-life Ronald Reagan was elected president.[45] By the early 1980s, *Roe v. Wade* had withstood challenges and threats, but a majority of public and private hospitals still refused to perform abortions.[46]

The right-to-life movement's success linking the right to abortion and the right to die spelled trouble for euthanasia advocates. They were dismayed (if not surprised) that, just as their activism was beginning to pay dividends in the form of living will legislation, they were being attacked by right-to-lifers who equated abortion and physician aid-in-dying.[47] In showdown after showdown, in state capital after state capital, SRD officials such as Rosoff, Helen Taussig, and Alice Mehling, testifying in favor of living will laws, faced off against Catholics and their allies in the New Right. The clash between pro-lifers and euthanasia advocates was most evident in California in 1976 when the first living will legislation, the California Natural Death Act, passed after considerable conflict and frantic compromises. Ultimately, both the medical profession and the state's Catholic hierarchy accepted a highly watered-down bill, but to right-to-life activists, their failure to stop the California Act only stiffened their resolve to stop living will legislation in other states.[48]

To euthanasia advocates with long memories, the confrontations with the right-to-life movement were reminiscent of the bitter battles with Catholics in the 1940s and 1950s. Euthanasia's opponents in the 1980s appeared just as dedicated, clever, and well-funded as ever.[49] Olive Ruth Russell was so worried about right-to-lifers that she feared they had actually infiltrated the CFD.[50] Some euthanasia proponents showed grudging admiration for their foes. "I must say," one euthanasia supporter admitted to Russell, "those people" in the antiabortion movement "hire very attractive and able speakers. I wouldn't mind if they would stick to the abortion issue, but at no extra expense they invariably sneak in the 'euthanasia dig.' "[51] The big difference between past and present was that, by the 1980s, euthanasia was conflated with the highly contentious abortion issue, an albatross that the right-to-die movement would just as soon have done without.

If the euthanasia movement faced robust opposition from the New Right, two developments on its radical wing also complicated matters. In 1976, the Japan Euthanasia Society was formed, and it invited similar organizations around the world to meet in Tokyo at the first International Euthanasia Conference. Delegates from five countries gathered in 1976 and issued the "Tokyo Declaration," which supported the legalization of an individual's right to die without suffering. Two years later delegates met in San Francisco at the Second International Euthanasia Conference. The success of these two conferences led in 1980 to the formation of the World Federation of Right-to-Die Societies, numbering twenty-seven organizations from eighteen countries, with the SRD's Sidney Rosoff elected its first president.

Virtually from the beginning of the World Federation, it was obvious that Europeans tended to be more sympathetic than Americans to active euthanasia. Testifying to the distinctive (and more moderate) nature of the American euthanasia movement and the different political culture it inhabited, CFD's board declined to join the international organization in 1980.[52] While the World Federation did not issue a common program, preferring to allow each organization to pursue its own objectives, it was clear that many in the international movement supported active euthanasia and assisted suicide. The antics of the English euthanasia group EXIT (formerly the Voluntary Euthanasia Society, to which name it would revert in 1981) deeply troubled the CFD board. In 1979, EXIT announced it would issue a "how-to" suicide manual (with a preface written by author Arthur Koestler) but soon canceled its plans when the predictable backlash occurred.[53] Then EXIT's general secretary and a volunteer were found guilty of aiding the deaths of several people, including some who were suffering from depression and alcoholism and were not terminally ill. Because EXIT had hosted the 1980 Oxford meeting of international right-to-die societies, the entire world organization was tarnished. The Oxford meeting, in McKinney's words, "did little to persuade our board that the Concern's goal to encourage reasoned and full consideration of complex issues in the whole field of euthanasia was shared by any but a handful" in the international movement.[54]

CFD later joined the World Federation in 1982, but its board was never comfortable about the affiliation. Its doubts about the international movement were reinforced in 1984 when, at the international right-to-die conference in Nice, France (the first to be open to the public), several speakers strongly endorsed the legalization of assisted suicide.[55] The radicalization of the international right-to-die movement helped to drive a wedge into the American movement, as events in the late 1980s would illustrate.

The formation of the Hemlock Society in 1980 drove that wedge even farther. Hemlock, the brainchild of British-born Derek Humphry, was a grassroots euthanasia organization with West Coast origins, a distinct departure from either CFD or the SRD. Its profound effect on the national right-to-die debate signaled that the leadership of the euthanasia movement in the 1980s and 1990s had ceased being monopolized by the Manhattan-based social elites that traditionally had spearheaded twentieth-century reform.

Humphry ranks as one of the preeminent pioneers of the American euthanasia movement. He began his career as a journalist and, after writing a book about helping his cancer-ridden first wife to die, he and his second wife, Ann Wickett, founded the Hemlock Society in Los Angeles in 1980.[56] Begun on a shoestring budget, Hemlock

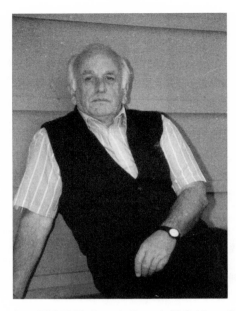

Derek Humphry. *ERGO! (Euthanasia Research & Guidance Organization).*

enjoyed a remarkable growth in the 1980s that rivaled anything the other U.S. organizations had achieved. By 1992, when Humphry retired from the group, Hemlock could boast eighty-six local chapters across the country, 57,000 members, and a newsletter, the *Hemlock Quarterly*, whose subscriber list had risen from 443 to close to 40,000.[57] What also distinguished Hemlock from CFD and the SRD was its official support for active euthanasia and assisted suicide. With Hemlock on the scene, the rest of the euthanasia movement felt pressured into taking a stand on these controversial issues. A casualty of this process was the SRD, which disappeared in 1990, leaving the agenda of the old ESA to be co-opted by first Hemlock, and then other, more radical groups in the 1990s.[58]

The founding of Hemlock occurred in the wake of the 1978 publication of Humphry's book, *Jean's Way*, his account of how he had assisted his first wife's death. As police investigated her death in England, Humphry relocated to the United States, where he was deluged with requests to travel and lecture about euthanasia. The avid interest of audiences in what he had to say convinced him to form an organization that, unlike CFD or the SRD, would officially support the decriminalization of assisted suicide and "active voluntary euthanasia for the terminally ill." Once Hemlock was up and running, he turned his attention to publishing the first American self-deliverance guide. Inspired by the Scottish EXIT's manual, Humphry wrote *Let Me Die Before I Wake*. *Let Me Die*, published in 1981, provided readers with information on nonviolent methods of suicide (such as drug dosages), interwoven with true stories of people who had attempted suicide. It became a best-seller, selling 62,000 copies within five years. In 1991 Humphry published *Final Exit*, a suicide guide with updated information. Meanwhile, Hemlock's headquarters had moved from California to Oregon, where in 1994 it helped to win the referendum on Measure 16, the Oregon Death With Dignity Act, permitting physicians to provide dying patients with lethal drugs for the purpose of suicide. By then, Humphry was a national celebrity.

However, the success of Humphry and Hemlock was compromised by embarrassing revelations about Humphry's personal life. In 1989 he left his second wife, Ann Wickett, shortly after she had undergone surgery for breast cancer. Their subsequent divorce was made messier by Wickett's allegations that her mother had not died willingly when Humphry had participated in the suicides of her own parents. In 1991 Wickett's cancer was in remission, but she was so depressed by Humphry's desertion and her unsuccessful lawsuit against Hemlock that one day she rode her horse into the Oregon woods and killed herself by taking a lethal dose of drugs. She left a suicide note, which turned out to be the last thing Humphry or Hemlock could have wanted. "There. You got what you wanted," she wrote to Humphry. "Ever since I was diagnosed as having cancer, you have done everything conceivable to precipitate my death." Even more damaging was that Wickett had sent a copy of the note to anti-euthanasia activist Rita Marker, with whom she had become friends after she and Humphry had separated. To Marker she wrote: "Rita: My final words to Derek. He is a killer. *I know.*" She then accused Humphry of actually suffocating his first wife, not simply supplying her with the medications to end her life.[59]

Humphry continues to insist that most of Wickett's troubles were due to what he calls her "borderline personality disorder."[60] Still, the emotional toll from the scandal likely helped persuade him to resign from Hemlock in 1992. Since then, he has devoted his time to writing, research, and lecturing. Humphry's goal remains first winning the legal right to assisted suicide, and then reaching "the second step" of active mercy killing.[61] In 2000 he invoked utilitarian reasons, reminiscent of those cited by the supporters of euthanasia in Potter's day, to suggest that there might be a "duty to die" on the part of America's elderly, who were "putting a strain on the health care system" by consuming dwindling funds that could be spent on other, healthier patients. In an era of cost containment in medical services, Humphry foresaw physician-assisted suicide as a solution to "the emotional, physical, and economic toll of the dying experience" on families, government, employers, hospitals, insurance companies and health care personnel.[62] Humphry and Hemlock have had a revolutionary impact on the right-to-die campaign in late-twentieth-century America, but his willingness to cite social and economic justifications for euthanasia was a throwback to earlier arguments in favor of mercy killing.

As Humphry worked to win support for euthanasia, other events and trends were helping to cultivate interest in physician-assisted suicide. In the 1980s, signs of a new suicide epidemic were beginning to emerge, especially among the elderly. The suicide rate among Americans over the age of sixty-five, after declining for four decades, rose during that decade. While comprising 13 percent of the population, the elderly were responsible for almost 20 percent of all suicides—the highest of any age group. Why senior citizens were choosing suicide in such numbers inevitably raised questions about the quality of their health care and the medical treatment of dying patients.[63]

The stunning appearance of AIDS, or acquired immune deficiency syndrome, also generated interest in euthanasia. First identified clinically in 1981, AIDS quickly became the leading killer of men between the ages of twenty-five and forty-four in the northeast United States, exacting a fearsome toll on the male homosexual population in particular. By the time the human immunodeficiency virus had been isolated and demonstrated in mid-1984 to be the cause of AIDS, thousands had already died. By 1988, 62,000 cases had been reported, more than half of whom had died. Those infected with the AIDS virus numbered in the hundreds of thousands. By the end of the 1980s, many Americans were still unaware of the actual ways AIDS was spread and who could contract it, but there were very few who had never heard of the disease.[64]

As is the case with America's elderly, AIDS patients are prone to suicide. A 1988 New York City study concluded that the relative risk of suicide in men with AIDS from the ages of twenty to fifty-nine was thirty-six times that of the general population. In the 1990s, AIDS patients made up "the vast majority of patients in hospices as well as those who seek the assistance of physicians in committing suicide." Physicians who treat AIDS patients likely help them to die more than any other medical specialty.[65]

If AIDS patients are more liable to choose medically assisted suicide, it is because they tend to die "hard deaths." The virus is an insidious organism that attacks and kills the body's immune cells before they have a chance to fight off disease. Although AIDS patients, normally well educated and affluent, have been able to raise impressive funds for research, medical science has not found a cure. As a result, people with AIDS normally die slowly and in great pain and discomfort from infections or cancer, often suffering from dementia, blindness, or disfiguring skin lesions. An AIDS diagnosis strikes many as a grotesque, horrific death sentence. Little wonder that the doubling of Hemlock's membership between 1988 and 1990 was partly due to an influx of AIDS patients.[66]

As the eighties wore on, both CFD and the SRD became closely associated with AIDS organizations, distributing living wills and providing AIDS patients with legal information about their rights, and as they did so they discovered how closely linked AIDS and euthanasia were. They learned of people such as Thomas Wirth, a forty-seven-year-old diagnosed with AIDS Related Complex (ARC), admitted to New York's Bellevue Hospital on 6 July 1987 in a stuporous, uncommunicative state. Prior to his admission, Wirth had granted power of attorney to a friend who protested the hospital's attempt to administer antibiotics in an effort to treat Wirth's toxoplasmosis, a parasitic infection responsible for his brain lesions. When the hospital persisted, Wirth's friend filed suit, but the New York State Supreme Court ruled that Bellevue was within its rights to order the treatment continued, even when Wirth did not immediately recover. The main problem stemmed from Wirth's living will, which did not make clear his wishes in such a case.[67]

As the SRD's director of legal services stated, Wirth's predicament "hammer[ed] home" the need for New York to pass living will legislation with provisions for the appointment of a proxy.[68] The problems Wirth experienced underlined how AIDS, perhaps more than any other condition, raised important questions about end-of-life treatment and the rights of patients who wished to die with dignity.

By focusing attention on the lengthy and pain-wracked deaths of AIDS patients, activists unavoidably highlighted the limited freedom Americans enjoyed when it came to exerting control over their deaths.

III.

By the late 1980s, the robust opposition of the right-to-life movement, the emergence of AIDS, and the radicalism of the Hemlock Society had helped to sharpen the differences between CFD and the SRD. CFD continued to move in a cautious direction, emphasizing education, information, counseling, and dialogue, rather than confrontation and legislation. The organization's stance reflected the views of interested parties who were wary about making the transition from endorsing passive to supporting active euthanasia. CFD continued to stress the complexity surrounding death with dignity rather than the need for broad policy solutions.

This clash in viewpoints between CFD and the SRD became obvious as early as 1981 when Don McKinney and Sidney Rosoff testified in Miami, Florida, before the President's Commission for the Study of Ethical Problems in Medicine and Biomedical and Behavioral Research. While Rosoff advocated legislation to permit the enforcement of patient wishes and end the threat of litigation to physicians or relatives, McKinney argued that fighting legislative battles over the enactment of living wills was divisive. He believed instead in more education of health care providers and the public about how patient decision-making was a right and how prolonging the dying process was futile. This open difference of opinion between CFD and the SRD increased the bitterness Rosoff and his group felt toward McKinney and drew attention to the fact that beneath the seemingly consensual rhetoric about death with dignity there were also grave disagreements dividing the American euthanasia movement.[69]

CFD's disagreement with the SRD showed up in its treatment of the Dax Cowart story. Overshadowed by *In re Quinlan*, the fate of Dax Cowart was no less central to an understanding of how Americans felt about euthanasia in the late twentieth century. Dax Cowart is the former Don Cowart who, as a twenty-five-year-old, was victimized by a horrendous accident on the night of 25 July 1973, near Kilgore, Texas. Dax and his father were appraising an eighty-acre property when their car's ignition sparked a pocket of propane gas, creating such a fireball that Cowart's father was killed. Dax, pinned helplessly inside the family car, was left with second- and third-degree burns covering his body, countless wounds from flying glass, and nothing but charred gristle for hands and the white of his exposed bones. While on the way to and undergoing treatment at Dallas's Parkland Memorial Hospital, Dax, in desperate agony, begged to be allowed to die, a wish he repeated over the many subsequent months of painful rehabilitation and reconstructive surgery. Seven years after the accident, he lay blind and crippled in a Galveston hospital, dependent on other people, unable to perform the simplest functions. Two suicide attempts had already failed, but he kept vowing to try again.[70]

In 1980, a freelance journalist talked CFD into doing a film documentary about Dax Cowart. The film, completed in 1984 and screened in cities such as Dallas and New York City, was a grim reminder that a freak accident could turn a handsome, bright rodeo rider and sports car driver into a helpless, distraught, disfigured, and suffering invalid. It was also a reminder that a patient's repeated wishes to withhold lifesaving treatment could be ignored by health care personnel. Unlike Karen Ann Quinlan's wishes, there was no mistaking what Dax said he wanted. As he discovered to his horror, the system was deaf to his pleas for a merciful death.

The Dax Cowart tale revealed that when it came to the question of who decides, there were no easy answers. In CFD's film, Dax appears as a more optimistic, much less suicidal person, who after years of grueling rehabilitation had married, attended law school, run a successful business, and, though still blind, walked three-quarters of a mile to work each day. In 1990, having just graduated from law school, he posed with his wife for a *Time* photographer.[71] His accident had actually given him a new identity. He had become a new person with a new name, no longer Donald but Dax, adopted because his poor hearing made it difficult to know whether people were talking to him or someone called John or Ron. Surgery, in the words of one eyewitness in 1982, had made him look "like pretty much your average blind person with blotchy skin."[72]

Although Dax Cowart continued to defend his right to refuse lifesaving treatment, he displayed a sardonic wit about his condition and expressed happiness with his job. His ordeal constituted a kind of template onto which people could project what they wanted to think. Either he was a poster boy for the right-to-die movement or he was a courageous fighter who overcame awesome odds to assert his right to live. Should his request to die have been honored? His life story seemed to say that, while there might be different answers to this question, it was difficult to choose the right one. Dax Cowart was a walking, talking, breathing example of what Donald McKinney and many in CFD had been preaching for years about the need for extreme caution when it came to euthanasia. "It is simplistic to say," McKinney remarked about Dax Cowart, "that the individual has a right to die. It is not that simple."[73]

McKinney's view that talking about a right to die was "simplistic" understandably strained relations between CFD and Derek Humphry's Hemlock Society. CFD's board took a dim view of EXIT's proposed suicide manual in 1980, and thus felt similarly about Humphry's 1981 *Let Me Die Before I Wake*. CFD's board believed that approval of suicide information guides would lead to people taking incorrect dosages, resulting in paralysis or massive brain damage without killing. According to CFD literature, such guides constituted "advocacy of suicide," and "erode the social consensus which currently supports efforts to improve care of the terminally ill and elderly."[74] In 1985 matters came to a head when a CFD official told the press about a distraught mother who had blamed her son's botched suicide on Humphry's book. This prompted a testy reply from Humphry, who asked McKinney why Hemlock had not been informed of the case before CFD talked to the press. "Isn't this a breach of conduct among fellow members of the World Federation of Right to Die Societies?" Humphry complained.[75]

As its interests steadily diverged from Hemlock's, CFD's position became so mainstream it was almost indistinguishable from that of the country's Roman Catholic Church. This similarity first surfaced at the presidential commission hearings in 1981, when McKinney found himself agreeing with Catholic spokespersons on living will legislation. Catholics argued that legislation was unnecessary because "the vast majority of patients are taken off life-supporting machines by following an ethical concept of an agreement between the doctors and families." They also invoked the "wedge theory," that living will legislation would lead to the legalization of active euthanasia. McKinney was more guarded in his comments, but he too pointed out that living wills might prove to be "a hindrance rather than a help to the providing of humane treatment and the honoring of a patient's wish."[76]

Imprecision of language and the failure to specify treatment under the widest range of circumstances possible were continuing problems with the living will, as the Thomas Wirth case demonstrated.[77] The promise of living wills was further tarnished in the 1980s as more and more health care experts recommended filling out a durable power of attorney (naming a surrogate to make decisions if one became incompetent), as either a supplement to a living will or as sufficient itself to ensure death with dignity. By the early 1990s, leading Americans such as Justice Sandra Day O'Connor of the U.S. Supreme Court and gerontologist and bioethicist Joanne Lynn had each stated that the better remedy than a living will was the durable power of attorney.[78] The fact that McKinney and CFD were lukewarm about living wills in the early 1980s, plus the presence of Catholic theologians and ethicists within CFD, drew the criticism from SRD hardliners that CFD had gone over to the other side.[79]

Despite these recriminations, there were signs of interest in a merger of CFD and the SRD as the 1980s wound down. To McKinney and many others in CFD, the 1980 split between the two organizations had been terribly unfortunate, and he blamed SRD board officials such as Rosoff and Ruth Proskauer Smith. In particular, pressure for a merger came from SRD physicians, most of whom expressed the historical resistance of their profession to formally approving physician-assisted suicide and active euthanasia. They were uneasy about statements uttered by individuals such as Joseph Fletcher, the SRD's president emeritus, who stated in 1989 that he wanted the group to "go down the road with Hemlock."[80] One of the SRD's physicians countered by saying, "I cannot endorse active euthanasia, nor would I want to be identified with the Hemlock Society. In fact, if the majority of the [SRD's] Board wish to subscribe to active euthanasia, I would resign from the Board."[81]

Thus, for a CFD-SRD merger to happen, some "heads" would "have to roll," predicted one SRD board member.[82] The "heads," it turns out, belonged to SRD members Fletcher, Sidney Rosoff, Ruth Smith, Joseph Fletcher, Olive Ruth Russell's former roommate Ruth Roettinger, Hugh Moore's widow Louise Van Vleck, and the lawyer Richard Wasserman. To many, they were the "representatives of the stressful period of the past," the chief reasons for the "bad blood" between CFD and the SRD in the late 1970s.[83] It was no coincidence they were also supporters of active euthanasia. By the end of the 1980s they were open to the idea of a merger, but they were united in their desire to thwart any attempt to water down the SRD's program. They sensed (correctly) that CFD was moving in a more conservative direction, while they were trying to inch the SRD toward advocacy of active euthanasia. Their eagerness to take the next leap in the history of the euthanasia movement ("to stretch ourselves" in Ruth Smith's words) led to a showdown that resulted in the end of the SRD itself.[84]

The first firm indication of efforts to get the SRD to "go down the road with Hemlock" began in the wake of the "Infant Doe" and "Baby Jane Doe" cases. "Infant Doe," born 9 April 1982 in Bloomington, Indiana, with Down syndrome and an obstructed esophagus, died six days later of starvation and dehydration when his parents refused to countenance the surgery and intravenous feeding that would have kept him alive. A year and a half later, "Baby Jane Doe" was born on Long Island, New York, with spina bifida, an abnormally small head, excess fluid in the brain, and a prolapsed rectum. Her parents first gave the go-ahead for surgery, but then quickly changed their minds, approving only feedings, antibiotics, and care of the exposed spinal sac. In April 1984 the parents changed their minds again and permitted surgeons to operate to relieve pressure on her brain. Four years later she was still alive, wheelchair-bound but talking and attending a school for the handicapped.[85]

The Indiana Supreme Court's decision not to rule in the Infant Doe case when prosecutors sought to have the court take custody of the child sparked strident condemnations from right-to-lifers, but it also emboldened some SRD members to declare their "commitment to the assurance and protection of the right of choice of the severely impaired newborn infant with respect to his/her death." Because an infant could not make this choice, the responsibility for medically informed decision-making ought to be invested in the baby's parents. The SRD never made this declaration public, but the consensus within the organization was that it simply extended a competent adult's right to refuse treatment to a defective infant. It also authorized a Haiselden-like form of involuntary euthanasia.[86]

Other signs of the SRD's radicalization became more evident at the group's annual meeting in late 1983 when Hemlock's Derek Humphry was the guest speaker, and in 1985 when it hosted Governor Richard Lamm of Colorado, who in 1984 had told a conference of lawyers that elderly Americans had "a duty to die, to get out of the way with our machines and our artificial hearts, so that our kids can build a reasonable life."[87] The 1984 Nice, France, international right-to-die meeting also turned the heads of some of the SRD's board who, inspired by European ideas, argued that once passive euthanasia was accepted, it was cruel and inhumane to deny those seeking death in an "easier and faster" manner the medical help in dying they requested. Some also agreed with Humphry that the "cost to society" justified the legalization of active euthanasia.[88] However, there were many within the SRD who still doubted the wisdom of openly advocating active euthanasia because it ran the risk of alienating moderate supporters, many of whom were "respondees to Dear Abby." As one SRD board member wondered, "will Abby still like us?" if the group endorsed physician-assisted suicide or active euthanasia.[89]

But the radicals would not let up the pressure. On 9 December 1986 Joseph Fletcher told the SRD that "the origin is the future." It was time to go "back to our original task as the Euthanasia Society of America perceived it." He urged the SRD to take a leadership role while joining Hemlock and other right-to-die societies around the world in backing active euthanasia and assisted suicide.[90] But he also wished to broaden active euthanasia by extending a "right to die" to people who were not actually dying and "helpless newborns or minors still too young to make any input into decisions about when to stop life-prolonging treatment."[91]

Reaction to Fletcher's speech endorsing voluntary and involuntary euthanasia was mixed at best. Predictably, it was music to the ears of Ruth Smith, who admitted that "board members groan every time I have quoted Joe [Fletcher] at board meetings."[92] Support for Fletcher's defense of assisted suicide also came from an SRD-sponsored conference at Harvard University in the fall of 1988. Six years earlier, in October 1982, the SRD had sponsored a physicians' conference, attended by euthanasia advocates Helen B. Taussig (who had written the foreword to Olive Ruth Russell's *Freedom to Die*); Peter Safar, professor of Resuscitation Medicine at the University of Pittsburgh; and Sidney Wanzer, an internist with Harvard Law School Health Services. The 1982 physicians' conference concluded that artificial feeding belonged to the same category of treatment as respirator support, and thus it was ethically permissible to discontinue such feeding if the patient's comfort was not affected by its removal.[93] In 1988, at the second physicians' conference, ten out of the twelve doctors agreed that it was "not immoral for a physician to assist the suicide of a rational, terminally ill person." Such a conclusion was not terribly surprising, given that four of the physicians who sided with the majority decision were members of the SRD board.[94]

But other SRD physicians and board members remained opposed to public declarations in favor of medically assisted suicide. This group, while expressing their support for assisted suicide under certain circumstances, were almost unanimous in their opposition to the SRD openly endorsing it. They rejected its legalization because, they thought, doing so would distract attention from the necessity to improve end-of-life care, such as pain management and emotional support of patients.[95] Privately, some believed the country was not "ready for euthanasia." There still appeared to be much work that had to be done among senior citizens who rarely had living wills, often not knowing what they were or how to execute them. This growing difference of opinion set the stage for an acrimonious showdown at a board meeting on 14 June 1989, when the SRD board voted not to endorse the decision of the ten physicians from the second Harvard conference.[96]

The Hemlock-like resolutions of the 1988 physicians' conference's proved to be the last straw for the moderates on the SRD board, convincing them that their future lay in a merger with the more conservative CFD. Actually, as early as January 1986, Don McKinney and SRD president Evan Collins Jr. had met to discuss such a CFD-SRD merger.[97] Talks truly began in earnest in early 1988 when SRD members started to see a merger as a way of purging troublesome radicals such as Rosoff, Joseph Fletcher, and Ruth Smith, and adopting CFD's "cautious" approach.[98] Things were made easier when CFD's board insisted that Rosoff be denied a board position with the new, amalgamated organization, tentatively titled the National Council on Death and Dying (NCDD).[99] When the merger appeared imminent, Rosoff, Smith, Wasserman, Joseph Fletcher, Ruth Roettinger, and Louise Van Vleck (widow of Hugh Moore) resorted to litigation in an attempt to block it. Thus, for the second time in ten years the two organizations headed to court to resolve their differences.

As had been the case in 1979–1980, financial considerations and personality issues played a part in the CFD-SRD merger. Both groups were running large deficits in 1989, and the prospect of combining their assets and centralizing their fund-raising efforts was attractive to many. Too, there was mounting impatience within the SRD with people such as Ruth Smith and Richard Wasserman, whose behavior others found to be "deeply offensive." One SRD member said Wasserman brought "an unwelcome tone" to negotiations with CFD and called him "representative of the worst of American lawyers." Another expressed her exasperation with Wasserman and Smith, who, by continually prodding the organization into adopting assisted suicide as official policy, "suggest[ed] that they were the only ones who stood for openness and that the rest of the Directors were scared people who wouldn't stand up for anything."[100]

But these tensions were nothing new to the history of the American euthanasia movement, which, like other cutting-edge social reform movements, attracted determined and independent-minded individuals who tended to believe they knew better than anyone else. The crux of the dispute remained the SRD's decision "not to take a public position in favor of physician-assisted suicide."[101] To Ruth Smith, this decision meant focusing on "the little Ohio lady in tennis shoes, who has not signed a Living Will. That is a micro, not a macro program. . . . It is a program we should be able to accomplish with our hands tied behind our backs." Far more important in her eyes was "the growing number of suicides—among the elderly—more with guns." Like Rosoff, Smith had reached the conclusion by the 1980s that these senior citizens needed active "assistance in dying" more than living wills.[102]

These differences over policy and philosophy set the stage for a tense series of meetings in early 1990, which resulted in Rosoff being voted off the board of directors for the new organization. Accusations of "fascism" and "hidden agendas" flew back and forth between supporters and opponents of the merger.[103] To the objectors, the SRD had been hijacked and, in Rosoff's words, a "fifty-year-old organization with a large national membership" had been "expunged." The issue was finally resolved in June 1991, with Ruth Smith being named to the NCDD's board of directors and Sidney Rosoff being granted the title of chairman emeritus. But Rosoff soon shifted his attention to Hemlock, and Smith resigned shortly after the merger, ending her forty-year-long association with the group.[104] An era stretching back to the days of the Euthanasia Society of America had come to an end.

Thus, the CFD-SRD negotiations culminated not so much in a merger as in a purge and a significant realignment of the euthanasia movement. Later in 1991, NCDD was renamed Choice in Dying, which became Partnership for Caring in 2000, a nonprofit organization dedicated to eliminating the suffering and improving the quality of life of dying persons and fostering communication about complex end-of-life decisions among individuals, their loved ones, and health care professionals. Like its predecessor CFD, Choice in Dying gradually distanced itself from the legislative arena and advocacy of physician-assisted suicide and active euthanasia, while promoting living wills and better care for the terminally ill. When Choice in Dying became Partnership for Caring, its board of directors took the legalization of physician-assisted suicide "off the table as an issue for policy development and political action."[105] Its evolution in the 1990s, based on its efforts to read the public's mood, indicated that its leadership believed American support for either assisted suicide or active euthanasia was a lot softer than the polling data indicated, and that Americans were more concerned about effective pain management and universal access to hospice and palliative care services.

In the meantime, one of the few remaining links to the ESA vanished when Joseph Fletcher died in 1991, but Hemlock and new organizations such as Compassion in Dying took up the old ESA agenda, seeking changes in state laws about active euthanasia or assisted suicide. Throughout the 1990s, as public interest in death and dying continued to mount against the backdrop of some of the most stunning events in the history of America's debate over euthanasia, they and not Choice in Dying would spearhead the campaign to legalize a right to die. By 2000, with more and more Americans asking themselves how they wanted to die, the nation's euthanasia movement had made considerable progress, leading one constitutional scholar to wonder whether the country was on the verge of a "social revolution." But, as Derek Humphry himself admitted at the end of 2001, the revolution was still a long way off.[106]

6

Conclusion: The 1990s and Beyond

The end of the Society for the Right to Die and the emergence of the new Choice in Dying in 1991 were just two in a dramatic sequence of events that, beginning in the late 1980s, marked a new chapter in a century-old saga. Throughout the 1990s, as opponents fought over physician-assisted suicide in America's courts, the political battleground shifted from the national arena to the state level. Promising opinion polls and the 1994 vote in Oregon in favor of the first law in America history permitting physician-assisted suicide appeared to give the euthanasia movement the decisive breakthrough that its activists had been dreaming about since the days of Charles Francis Potter.[1]

But there were also signs that Americans' wariness about legalizing euthanasia had not changed much, even if support for its clandestine practice was at an all-time high. The Oregon victory was followed by referendum defeats in Michigan and Maine, and a 1997 U.S. Supreme Court ruling that denied a constitutional right to physician-assisted suicide. As the twenty-first century dawned, euthanasia proponents faced the daunting prospect of having to fight many more hotly contested political battles in other states against an opposition that was no longer confined solely to the churches and the pro-life movement. As Derek Humphry conceded in 2001, the struggle for legalized euthanasia in America is "going to be a very long battle. This is still a religious country."[2] While much had changed since the days of Charles Potter, much had remained the same.

I.

While Concern for Dying and the Society for the Right to Die were engaged in their second bitter civil war within a decade, many Americans were impatiently awaiting a U.S. Supreme Court ruling on a death with dignity case that rivaled the legal wrangle over Karen Ann Quinlan. The story had begun one night in 1983, when the car of twenty-five-year-old Nancy Cruzan slid off an icy Missouri road. The ensuing crash threw her out of the car and left her breathless and without a pulse. Minutes later, paramedics revived her heartbeat and respiration, but Cruzan never regained consciousness. She spent the next seven years of her life in a permanent vegetative state, able to breathe but kept alive by a feeding tube; she was one of 10,000 Americans in a similar predicament.[3]

When the Missouri Supreme Court refused to grant her parents' request to withdraw her feeding tube, stating that without a living will Nancy Cruzan's real wishes were unclear, the case went to the U.S. Supreme Court, the first time the court agreed to hear a right-to-die case. In 1990 the justices ruled that a competent person had a constitutionally protected right to refuse any medical treatment, but it upheld Missouri's right to insist on clear and convincing evidence of the wishes of patients who did not have decision-making capacity before such treatment was discontinued. In the ruling's aftermath, the Cruzans' lawyer went back to court with new evidence of Nancy's prior wishes, and this time Missouri withdrew from the case, paving the way for her parents to finally remove the controversial feeding tube. Twelve days later, on 26 December 1990, Nancy Cruzan died at the age of thirty-three, seven years after being thrown from her car. But the Cruzans' suffering did not end, even with Nancy's death. In 1996 her father, Joe, hanged himself in the family's carport.[4]

The U.S. Supreme Court ruling in the Cruzan case, like its ruling seven years later on physician-assisted suicide, was a fittingly opaque decision for an issue that was just "not that simple," in Donald McKinney's words. The five-to-four split among the justices demonstrated how by the 1990s the right to die had become an exceedingly complex matter. Different interpretations of *Cruzan v. Missouri Director, Department of Health* abounded. Unusually, there were four separate written opinions among the justices, a reflection of the conflicting emotions it aroused.[5]

The Society for the Right to Die submitted an *amicus curiae* (friend of the court) brief in the Cruzan case and worked closely with the Cruzans, providing them with counseling and putting them in touch with a lawyer to represent them. The SRD castigated the Missouri Supreme Court's decision to overrule the lower court finding that Nancy Cruzan should be allowed to die. Rose Gasner, the SRD's director of legal services, remarked that the state supreme court made her "ashamed to be a lawyer," but she applauded the Missouri Department of Health's decision that it would not stand in Cruzan's parents' way to remove her life support. According to Gasner, who with Sidney Rosoff and Richard Wasserman wrote the SRD brief, no state interest outweighed Nancy Cruzan's constitutional and common law right to refuse the continuation of artificial feeding, nor—significantly—did she forfeit this right because of her incompetence. "A surrogate decision-maker, including a guardian, must be permitted to exercise these rights," the SRD brief stated. The U.S. Supreme Court's ruling that individuals did enjoy such a right as long as there was clear and convincing evidence of the person's wishes caused *Boston Globe* columnist Ellen Goodman to remark: "The Living Will. Don't leave home without it."[6]

Euthanasia activists, including Derek Humphry and many in the SRD, optimistically interpreted *Cruzan v. Missouri Director, Department of Health* as a constitutional recognition of the right to die, and thus a giant legal step closer to a similar recognition of a right to assisted suicide.[7] Equally hopeful news for Humphry and Hemlock came from a series of stunning events that in the late 1980s and early 1990s propelled the right-to-die debate to the center of national attention. The first shock came in 1988 when an anonymous article in the *Journal of the American Medical Association*, titled "It's Over, Debbie," told of how a gynecology resident in a large American private hospital had injected a patient suffering from painful ovarian cancer with an overdose of morphine sulphate. Called to her bedside in the middle of the night, the resident claimed she told him "Let's get this over with," whereupon he administered the lethal dose.[8]

Many condemned the resident for what he had done, arguing that, because he did not know the patient and had not talked to her or consulted with other physicians, he had essentially flouted all the safeguards euthanasia advocates normally proposed. Others attacked the *JAMA* for publishing the article in the first place, and some, such as columnist Charles Krauthammer, thought it was all a hoax, alleging that even extreme euthanasia proponents would not have killed in this way.[9] Hemlock's Derek Humphry disapproved of the young doctor's methods, though he acknowledged his compassion. Others expressed relief that the "Debbie" article had forced the fact that doctors did perform active euthanasia out into the open. "It makes no sense to hide our heads in the sand," one physician advised the *JAMA*'s readers.[10]

The controversy that greeted the publication of the "Debbie" story intensified in 1990 when Jack Kevorkian helped Janet Adkins to die. Before that date, Kevorkian had been an obscure pathologist, whose unconventional ideas about experimenting on dying, condemned criminals had caused his ostracism from the medical profession. Ever the maverick, Kevorkian believed in euthanasia on demand, provided by doctors without government regulation, for both mentally competent and incompetent patients.[11] Adkins, a Hemlock Society member, had seen Kevorkian on the *Donahue* television program and heard about Kevorkian's "mercitron," the suicide machine he had built. In June 1990, recently diagnosed with Alzheimer's disease, she agreed to meet Kevorkian in Michigan, where there was then no law against assisted suicide, and it was there, in the retired pathologist's rusty Volkswagen van, that she died.[12]

When news of Adkins's death broke, vigorous condemnation of Kevorkian quickly ensued. The Michigan Board of Medicine suspended his medical license in 1991, and in 1992 the state of Michigan passed a law making assisted suicide a felony. Like "Debbie"'s death, Adkins's suicide at Kevorkian's hands had not been approved by other physicians, nor had Kevorkian known Adkins for long or her full clinical history. Adkins had not been dying, and, although apparently perfectly sane, had never been screened by a psychiatrist.[13] Nonetheless, the Hemlock Society called Kevorkian a "brave pioneer," and he enjoyed the staunch support of the founder of

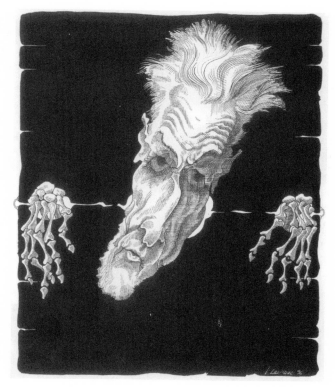

Drawing of Jack Kevorkian by Vint Lawrence. *J. Vinton Lawrence.*

Michigan's Hemlock chapter.[14] Derek Humphry "respected Kevorkian's courage and determination," while acknowledging that "they were on separate paths to the same goal: Kevorkian's to alter the medical profession's attitude, and Hemlock's to change the law." Officially, Hemlock preferred laws regulating assisted suicide to Kevorkian's actions, but there was a great deal of residual sympathy among its members for the services he provided to patients.[15]

After a brief court appearance, during which the charges against him were dismissed, Kevorkian over the next eight years went on to help at least ninety-three people die, sixty-three of them women.[16] During that same period, three different juries refused to indict him, suggesting that public opinion was behind him. But appearances were deceptive. News of Kevorkian's actions likely helped to scuttle a major campaign in Washington State to legalize "physician-aid-in-dying" in 1991. Washington State's Initiative 119 was actually the second of three state ballot initiatives in the early 1990s (Michigan in 1998 and Maine in 2000 are the others) that sought the legalization of physician-assisted suicide through referenda. California, Washington, and Oregon were targeted by euthanasia activists because most of the right-to-die groups were headquartered on the West Coast by the early 1990s, including Hemlock, Compassion in Dying, Americans for Death With Dignity, and ERGO! The area is also where the New Age movement, with its positive affirmation of death as a meaningful experience, is most strongly rooted.[17] However, when the votes were counted in 1991, Washington's Initiative 119 had been defeated, 53.6 percent to 46.4 percent.[18]

The trend toward populist efforts such as Initiative 119 had begun in 1986 when Robert Risley formed Americans Against Human Suffering (AAHS), a nonprofit organization and the "political wing" of Hemlock. The AAHS mission was to go state by state, trying to change the laws to permit physician-assisted suicide, and it identified California as the first place to get a right-to-die initiative on the ballot.[19] After failing in California to obtain the required number of signatures in 1988, three years later the campaign shifted to Washington State where a new figure on the right-to-die scene, Unitarian minister Ralph Mero, spearheaded the crusade. Originally, Mero had helped to found Washington State's Hemlock chapter, drawn to the organization after watching his father's protracted illness and subsequent death and his brother-in-law die of AIDS. He later rebelled against Hemlock's then policy of refusing to help people find the assistance they needed in dying, cofounding Compassion in Dying in 1993.[20] In 1990 Mero formed Washington Citizens for Death With Dignity (WCDD), which gathered the necessary signatures for Initiative 119. He and WCCD managed to cobble together a broad coalition of groups, some recent recruits to the euthanasia cause such as AIDS organizations, and others with links to the movement dating back decades, including the Humanists and the Unitarian Universalist Association.

Ignoring advice from Humphry and other Hemlock personnel, Mero crafted a vaguely worded initiative with few explicit safeguards; at first this appeared to be no liability as early indications pointed to a victory for the 119 side. The 119 campaigners were heartened by Congress's 1991 Patient Self-Determination Act, which ordered all hospitals, hospices, and nursing homes participating in Medicare and Medicaid programs to inform patients of their right not only to accept or refuse medical treatment but also execute a living will. The 119 side was likewise gratified to hear that Derek Humphry's *Final Exit* had vaulted to the top of the best-seller list, and that right-to-die activists were preparing to launch initiatives similar to Mero's 119 in other states.[21]

However, about two months before Washingtonians went to the polls, the anti-119 forces staged a remarkable rally that ultimately swept them to victory. They were aided when the public learned in the days before the vote that Kevorkian had just helped two more women die, frightening many into believing that 119 would lead to Kevorkian-like practices. More unwelcome publicity for the pro-119 forces was the press coverage of Ann Wickett's death, which 119 opponents exploited to drive home the message that the Wicketts of the world would be the victims of such a law.

The news coming out of the Netherlands in 1991 was also damaging to 119 supporters, who insisted that permitting euthanasia would not result in abuses. Until 2001, when the Netherlands officially legalized physician-assisted suicide and voluntary active euthanasia, the Dutch Penal Code outlawed both practices. However, a series of decisions beginning in the 1970s in effect had decriminalized them and conferred immunity from prosecution on doctors who performed them. In 1990 the Netherlands government appointed a commission to examine how euthanasia was actually being practiced in that country. The results, in what was called the Remmelink Report, surprised the commission itself, which had assumed that euthanasia was rare and controlled by the existing guidelines. The Remmelink Report of 1991 revealed that nonvoluntary euthanasia had occurred in a noticeable number of cases, amounting to as many as 1.6 percent of all deaths in the Netherlands. A follow-up study in 1995 found that underreporting of euthanasia by Dutch physicians continued to be a serious problem, and the number of mercy killings in which explicit consent had not been obtained was unacceptably high. To critics of euthanasia, the Dutch data were proof that if a right to die became reality it would be difficult to ensure that personal consent always preceded mercy killing. Opponents of the Netherlands law contended that in the United States, without the Dutch universal health care system, legalized euthanasia would be used to rid hospitals and nursing homes of difficult or inconvenient patients.[22]

Nor did it help the Initiative 119 cause that most Washington State physicians opposed it. The Washington State Medical Association and a group called Washington Physicians Against 119 defended the orthodox viewpoint that doctors wanted to care for their patients, "not kill them." The American Medical Association also mailed thousands of brochures containing anti-119 information.[23] But probably the most decisive factor in the defeat of Washington's Initiative 119 was the massive amount of money spent by pro-life organizations and institutions, notably the Roman Catholic Church. Public figures such as former Surgeon General C. Everett Koop as well as Catholic clerics and groups from across the nation, hammered away at the Washington initiative, claiming it was the first step toward legalizing a process that would see people being pressured to die for financial and social reasons. John Cardinal O'Connor, Archbishop of New York, compared the initiative with "the small beginnings" of Nazi genocide during World War II.[24] The vote count confirmed that people responded to this rhetoric, transforming the Washington campaign into yet another tough lesson in tactics for the euthanasia movement.

Making public appearances in favor of the Washington "physician-aid-in-dying" law was the Rochester, New York, physician Timothy Quill, who had almost overnight became a leading spokesperson for the right-to-die movement. At the height of the Initiative 119 campaign, a grand jury refused to indict the forty-three-year-old Quill, who, in 1990, had announced in a groundbreaking *New England Journal of Medicine* article that "Diane," a longtime patient of his suffering from painful leukemia, had killed herself by taking lethal drugs he had prescribed for her.[25] Quill had concluded from his training and experience treating terminally ill patients that even in the best of hospice care there were still "pretty tough deaths." He decided to go public with the "Diane" case because he believed there was a genuine need to "deepen the discussion [about dying] within the profession." Quill urged the legalization of assisted suicide, but only to safeguard a process that was going on anyway in American medicine and only as a last resort when the best palliative care failed. He was willing to go all the way to the U.S. Supreme Court, which in 1997 heard arguments about a 1994 complaint filed by Quill and five others, challenging New York State's penal law prohibiting assisted suicide.[26]

Bespectacled, bearded, balding, and soft-spoken, Quill was the polar opposite of the often irascible and abrasive Kevorkian, and as a physician he exuded a professional authority that Derek Humphry never enjoyed. Quill's unhurried, empathetic, and questioning approach to euthanasia has won the admiration of many Americans, including the well-known physician and author Sherwin Nuland.[27]

All the same, Quill's intervention in the Washington State campaign did not make much of a difference, nor did his lobbying in 1992 when Californians failed to ratify an initiative similar to Washington's 119. Leading the California Proposition 161 forces was AAHS founder Robert Risley and his renamed Californians Against Human Suffering. Once again, early polls showed the right-to-die movement out in front with a substantial lead, but as in Washington, the lead steadily dwindled when 161's opponents (chiefly the Catholic Church) began spending freely on advertising. Those urging a "no" vote stressed that no matter how heartrending individual cases were, a law on assisted suicide would inevitably lead to abuses. The outcome, a 54 to 46 percent victory for the anti-161 side, demonstrated that euthanasia's enemies were masters at all-out, no-holds-barred political campaigning, what Humphry later dubbed "pure political theater."[28]

Undaunted and more savvy, right-to-die proponents trained their sights on Oregon, Humphry's home state. Hemlock of Oregon formed its own political action committee, Oregon Right to Die (ORTD), to launch and lead the initiative, called Measure 16. Oregon's political culture, emphasizing libertarianism, progressive populism, and the lowest rate of churchgoing of all the states in America, proved to be key. In 1994, the Oregon Death With Dignity Act was passed by a 51 to 49 percent margin.

As in California and Washington State, the right-to-die forces started with a hefty lead in the opinion polls, but history appeared to be repeating itself when, as the campaign progressed, the anti-Measure 16 side started to make headway. The American Medical Association opposed the initiative and, as it had done in the other two states, the Catholic Church entered the fray with its considerable financial clout, backed by a coalition of Mormon, Episcopal, Lutheran, Baptist, and Evangelical organizations. But ORTD cleverly managed to turn the entire debate into "a battle between rigid religionists and compassionate rationalists," between one group of Americans seeking to impose their moral values on another group, echoing what Protestants and Other Americans United for the Separation of Church and State had contended back in the 1940s. As one pro-Measure 16 radio ad warned, "there are just some people who believe they have a divine right to control other people's lives, and they'd better back off because it's none of their business."[29] This strategy of reducing the debate over Measure 16 into a conflict between religion and secular choice worked, but it neatly sidestepped the fact that euthanasia historically enjoyed the support of the Unitarian Universalist church, Ethical Culture, and the American Humanist Association, all groups that (at least initially) claimed to be religious.

Pro-Measure 16 activists also capitalized on the perception that their euthanasia law was more conservative than the California initiative, which would have allowed doctors to administer lethal injections to their dying patients. The Oregon statute permitted physicians to prescribe only oral medications and came with numerous safeguards. In the initial planning stages, Derek Humphry and others had opposed limiting Measure 16 this way, and Humphry to this day believes that victory would have been won even if the law included voluntary active euthanasia.[30] When he was unable to persuade fellow activists to broaden the law, he decided to keep his thoughts to himself throughout the campaign, but once the victory had been won he stated his "doubts [about] the effectiveness of the new Oregon law." Stressing that suicides often miscarry, he contended that the law would work only "if in every instance a doctor is standing by to administer the coup de grace if necessary." Humphry asserts he is "in this movement for the long haul," and will not stop until voluntary active euthanasia, virtually on demand, is legalized.[31]

The Oregon law remained in legal limbo for another three years, until September 1997 when the U.S. Supreme Court declined to hear an appeal of a lower court ruling that upheld the law. But Oregonians who wished to take advantage of the law remained frustrated as the decade drew to a close. Opponents of physician-assisted suicide in Congress tried to render Oregon's statute toothless by passing a bill that amended the federal Controlled Substances Act, outlawing the use of narcotics to cause death. The bill not only deterred Oregon doctors from helping their patients die, it also made them fear that their aggressive attempts to alleviate patients' pain might lead to prosecution. These fears became all too real when in late 2001 Attorney General John Ashcroft ordered federal drug enforcement agents to crack down on doctors who prescribed lethal drugs to their dying patients. A federal judge in Oregon extended a restraining order against Ashcroft's directive, making assisted suicide legal again, pending a trial in 2002. Naturally, right-to-die proponents hope the courts will rule in their favor, but even if Ashcroft fails in his effort to thwart Oregon's law, there are few signs that the issue will become any less contested in coming years.[32]

Meanwhile, as the Oregon statute wound its way through the courts, the euthanasia movement's fortunes were no rosier on another front. Two challenges to New York State's and Washington State's prohibitions against physician-assisted suicide reached the federal Supreme Court in 1997. Timothy Quill, along with two other physicians and three mentally competent patients, challenged the New York State penal law that states that a person who intentionally helps another person commit suicide is guilty of manslaughter in the second degree. In June 1997 the court upheld both states' laws against assisted suicide and found no constitutional basis for a right to die in the "equal protection" Fourteenth Amendment, as had two lower appeals courts. A glimmer of hope for right-to-die activists could be found in the justices' refusal to bar states from legalizing euthanasia, shifting the debate from federal courts to the states, but the court's ruling "abruptly ended" the debate over a constitutional right to physician-assisted suicide.[33] The justices had not closed the door on the plaintiffs and their supporters completely, but only the sunniest of optimists could believe that either *Vacco v. Quill* or *Washington v. Glucksberg* brought them much closer to the *Roe v. Wade*-like triumph they had long sought.[34]

The Supreme Court's decision was followed by initiatives in Michigan (1998) and Maine (2000), both losses for the euthanasia movement. The two votes underlined the historically contingent nature of the struggle over the right to die in America as well as the chronic difficulties the movement faced over the course of the twentieth century. The defeat in Michigan was shocking, given the emphatic results when Oregonians went back to the polls in 1997 and voted 60 to 40 percent to keep their 1994 Death With Dignity Act. The defeat in Maine was much narrower, 51.5 to 48.5 percent. However, to the *American Medical News*, "that physician-assisted suicide measures fail at all ... is remarkable." The pitch to voters from euthanasia supporters relentlessly plays "the compassion card" and invariably stresses how such a law widens the scope of personal freedom.[35] The Maine and Michigan results may be some of the first indications that Americans are becoming increasingly skeptical about the social consequences of an "unvanquished individualism," "the beginnings of a historically inevitable, and perhaps not entirely unhealthy, reaction against the pathologies of the unencumbered self."[36] As Americans worry about the fraying of the national fabric and rethink the accepted meanings of community, they wonder whether or not expanding the notion of individual autonomy to include such things as a right to physician-assisted suicide "would be unwise and dangerous public policy." The "appeal to autonomy," so cherished in American society, should never be the paramount value when devising policy to cover death and dying, as the important New York State Task Force on Life and the Law concluded in 1994. In the words of Justice Anthony Kennedy in 1997 (citing the New York State Task Force), the individual autonomy that euthanasia advocates seek is "illusory" and in the long run will actually "diminish choices, not increase them."[37]

The failure of Michigan and Maine voters to respond positively to appeals invoking "compassion" and personal freedom signaled that the momentarily high hopes for a domino effect after the victory in Oregon were beginning to fade by the early twenty-first century. At the time of the 1997 second vote in Oregon, Barbara Coombs Lee, executive director of the pro-euthanasia Compassion in Dying, hailed the results as "a turning-point for the death with dignity movement," and others called the vote "a good indicator of where America may be headed."[38] But as Derek Humphry freely admits, defeat in Oregon inspired the Christian Right to organize more effectively and fight the Maine and Michigan battles all the more aggressively.[39] Opposition to legalized physician-assisted suicide has also broadened to include people and groups beyond the boundaries of right-to-life organizations and the Christian Right, most notably the New York State Task Force on Life and the Law, whose 1994 *When Death Is Sought* report was a landmark event in the history of America's debate over euthanasia.

The vote counts in Washington, California, Michigan, and Maine are indeed curious when opinion polls in the 1990s consistently tell analysts that clear majorities of Americans favor the freedom to choose assisted suicide. Gallup surveys indicate that support for active voluntary euthanasia has grown from 37 percent in 1947 to 69 percent in 1990. Poll data in 1995 also reveal that support for physician-assisted suicide is growing among American physicians, and that four out of five American doctors working in adult intensive care units around the country have withheld or withdrawn treatment they felt was futile, sometimes without informing family members and over relatives' objections.[40] Like Derek Humphry and Faye Girsh, executive director of Hemlock Society, USA, Timothy Quill objects to the hypocrisy of outlawing physician-assisted suicide, while permitting the practice of physicians drugging pain-wracked dying patients into comas and then removing hydration and nutrition so the patients die of starvation and dehydration, in what is called "terminal sedation."[41] With the Netherlands enacting laws permitting physician-assisted suicide, and prospects for similar victories in Belgium and Luxembourg, it remains to be seen how America will resist the temptation to follow international trends.

However, poll numbers in the United States are deceptive. Americans endorse a generalized and abstract right to die, but when pollsters ask questions relating to specific medical situations, public support declines. This is particularly true about voluntary active euthanasia, which Americans tend to tolerate but only when the patient is in unremitting pain and definitely terminally ill.[42] In the final analysis, as bioethicist Ezekiel Emanuel argues, a "rule of thirds" dominates polling data regarding euthanasia: a third of Americans endorse legalization under a wide variety of circumstances, a third oppose it under any circumstances, and a third support it in isolated cases but oppose it under most circumstances. Support for either active euthanasia or physician-assisted suicide is neither strong nor deep.[43] As the legal expert and anti-euthanasia warhorse Yale Kamisar declared in 2002, "it is much easier to sell the basic notion of assisted suicide than to sell a complex statue making the idea law."[44] As regrettable as terminal sedation is, there is no evidence that public opinion prefers the alternative of changing professional standards and the law to authorize euthanasia, thus running the risk of any further erosion of society's respect for life. According to Donald McKinney, a member of the New York State Task Force on Life and the Law, "a deliberate act to assist someone in taking his/her life—however merciful the intent—should not be sanctioned by law. Rather it should be left a private act, with society able to be called in to judgment when and if the motive should be impugned. This is not a neat and precise system of justice to be sure, but one that continues to afford the least possibility of abuse."[45]

The fallout from September 11 may also strengthen this less than "neat and precise" compromise, which most Americans appear to sanction at the beginning of the twenty-first century. One of the strongest elements in the thinking of euthanasia advocates is the desire for self-determination, the urge of individuals to choose a course of action that is both free from constraints imposed by others and in accordance with personal values. But as historian Peter Filene argues, there is a "desperate desire for control" beneath the surface of such sentiments, a wish that even a living will often fails to realize, as the case of AIDS victim Thomas Wirth illustrated. The many varieties of death human beings experience can rarely be made dignified, and the terrorist attacks of September 11 showed the fiction underlying even the most careful plans for a medically managed death. Ultimately, the concepts of death with dignity and choice in dying may have little meaning in a world where one's death can be so fortuitous and unanticipated, so beyond individual control.[46] Such concepts may be myths masquerading as democratic ideals.

The impasse the euthanasia movement has reached in the early twenty-first century may only be temporary, and the floodgates dreaded by the anti-euthanasia forces may swing wide open at some point in the not too distant future. The fortunes of the euthanasia movement have been firmly embedded in the twists and turns of American history, and history undoubtedly has several more in store. But the sobering and plain lesson of the last three decades for euthanasia advocates is that more than favorable polls are necessary before right-to-die campaigners can realistically hope for the widespread decriminalization of physician-assisted suicide, much less active voluntary euthanasia. They find themselves in roughly the same position they've occupied at prior junctures in their history, confronted with the prospect that they might have misjudged the country's popular mood, wondering indeed if they had alienated "Dear Abby" and "the little old Ohio ladies in tennis shoes."

Whatever the fate of the euthanasia movement, there is no denying how resourceful its advocates have been in crafting their message to fit America's changing times. But in other respects, that message has remained remarkably consistent. Though they may not know it, today's defenders of the right to die often echo the justifications of euthanasia first uttered by people such as Robert Ingersoll and Felix Adler, and later offered by Charles Francis Potter, Charlotte Perkins Gilman, Olive Ruth Russell, Florence Clothier, and Walter Sackett. Their deep commitment to relieve human suffering has led them to advocate policies that at first glance seem to extend inalienable and overdue rights to individuals who have been denied them by groups that wish to impose their values on the rest of society. However, the history of euthanasia in America suggests this is a simplistic diagnosis of a gravely complex social, political, economic, and cultural matter. Talk of a right to die raises the troubling questions: once legalized for the dying, who can be denied such a right? The chronically ill, but not dying? Pain-free patients who nonetheless feel their medical conditions leave them with no quality of life? Depressed teenagers? The mentally ill? Handicapped children whose parents wish them dead? Infants with severe disabilities? Where does the freedom to die end and the duty to die begin? The history of euthanasia in America reminds us that, despite a century of intensive debate and passionate political battles, these questions remain largely unanswered.

Abbreviations Used in Notes

ABCL American Birth Control League
ACLU American Civil Liberties Union
AHA American Humanist Association
AVS Association for Voluntary Sterilization
BC Brock Chisholm Papers, National Archives of Canada, Ottawa, Ontario
CFD Concern for Dying
CID Choice in Dying
CMAC Voluntary Euthanasia Society Records, Contemporary Medical Archives Center, Wellcome Institute for the History of Medicine, London
EEC Euthanasia Educational Council
EEF Euthanasia Educational Fund
ESA Euthanasia Society of America
FC Florence Clothier Papers, Schlesinger Library, Radcliffe College, Cambridge, Mass.
HBAA Human Betterment Association of America
HK Horace Kallen Papers, American Jewish Archives, Cincinnati, Ohio

HM	Hugh Moore Fund Collection, Seeley G. Mudd Library, Princeton University
ICP	Inez Celia Philbrick Papers, Nebraska State Historical Library, Lincoln
JDR	John D. Rockefeller 3rd Papers, Rockefeller Archive Center, Tarrytown, N.Y.
MSP	Margaret Sanger Papers, *Collected Documents*
NAC	Olive Ruth Russell Papers, National Archives of Canada, Ottawa, Ontario
NSLE	National Society for the Legalization of Euthanasia
POAU	Protestants and Other Americans United for Separation of Church and State
PFC	Partnership for Caring, Inc., Records, Lewis Associates, Baltimore, Md.
PPFA	Planned Parenthood Federation of America
RLD	Robert Latou Dickinson Papers, Francis Countway Library, Rare Books Department, Harvard University Medical School, Boston
RPS	Ruth Proskauer Papers, Schlesinger Library, Radcliffe Institute, Harvard University
SRD	Society for the Right to Die
SWHA	EngenderHealth Records, Social Welfare History Archives, University of Minnesota, Minneapolis
VELS	Voluntary Euthanasia Legislation Society
VES	Voluntary Euthanasia Society

Notes

Introduction

1. The New York State Task Force on Life and the Law, *When Death Is Sought,* 100–101.
2. Proctor, *The Nazi War on Cancer,* 270–71.
3. Critchlow, *Intended Consequences.* 9.
4. In *Intended Consequences,* Donald Critchlow has said similar things about the family planning movement in twentieth-century America. Critchlow's book is a careful examination of the way concerns over population control, birth control, and abortion intersected to shape federal family planning policy.
5. Nuland, *How We Die,* xvi–xvii.
6. Pernick, *The Black Stork,* 3–114.

Chapter 1

1. McKim, *Heredity and Human Progress,* 188–89, 190–91, 193, 213, 254, 259. His emphasis.
2. Fye, "Active Euthanasia: An Historical Survey of Its Conceptual Origins and Introduction into Medical Thought," 492–502, quote on 492; Hudson, "The Many Faces of Euthanasia," 102–7.

3. America seemed to be in "perpetual transition," with growing numbers of intellectuals and social scientists questioning its moral pieties and its inherited conventions. See Dorothy Ross, "Modernist Social Science in the Land of the New/Old," in Ross, ed., *Modernist Impulses in the Human Sciences, 1870–1930,* 183–84.

4. Graham, *The Great Campaigns Reform.* See also Hays, *Conservation and the Gospel of Efficiency.*

5. The Christian Fundamentalist movement was launched in 1910, and between 1916 and 1926 church membership across the country actually rose a striking 31 percent. Robert Dallek, "Modernizing the Republic, 1920 to the Present," in Bailyn et al., eds., *The Great Republic,* 713.

6. Conkin, *When All the Gods Trembled,* 58–59.

7. In 1972, the Central Conference of American Rabbis stated that "the Jewish ideal of sanctity of human life and the supreme value of the individual soul would suffer incalculable harm if, contrary to the moral law, men were at liberty to determine the conditions under which they might put an end to their own lives and the lives of other men." Muriel Franzblau to Olive Ruth Russell, 8 November 1972, NAC, MG31-K13, vol. 2, file 18. As late as 1997 even Reform Judaism, the most liberal and progressive of all the branches of Judaism, refused to declare that euthanasia was consistent with Jewish values. Larson and Amundsen, *A Different Death,* 51–54.

8. Little is known of the oath's origins, though it likely dates from between the fifth and third centuries B.C. Porter, *The Greatest Benefit to Mankind,* 62; Gourevitch, "Suicide Among the Sick in Classical Antiquity," 501–18. See also Larson and Amundsen, *A Different Death,* 31–35.

9. While examples of suicide as martyrdom abound in Judaic literature, the circumstances under which martyrs killed themselves are so radically different from those of terminally or seriously ill patients that they can in no way be interpreted as justifications for medical euthanasia or physician-assisted suicide. In fact, in the Old Testament there are no instances of people committing suicide or requesting others to assist them in suicide to put an end to illness-induced suffering. Larson and Amundsen, *A Different Death,* 36–38.

10. This generalization about Christian attitudes even applied to the early Christian martyrs. None of them desired death as a release from physical or mental suffering but accepted death only in imitation of Christ at the hands of a persecuting state. Larson and Amundsen, *A Different Death,* 38–60.

11. Larson and Amundsen, *A Different Death,* 137, 140. See also Minois, *History of Suicide,* 33, 35.

12. Ironically, it was a Catholic martyr, Sir Thomas More, who in *Utopia* (1516) came closest of all his contemporaries to endorsing active euthanasia, although the term had not yet been coined. More, lord chancellor to Henry VIII of England, was beheaded in 1535 for refusing to swear allegiance to his king as head of the reformed English church. In 1935 Pope Pius XI canonized More, an act that

would later be cited gleefully by twentieth-century euthanasia advocates in their efforts to discredit Catholic opposition to mercy killing. Modern-day euthanasiasts, however, ignore the fact that no one is sure what in *Utopia* More intended to be taken seriously. In *Utopia*, More foresaw a state in which those suffering from incurable and painful diseases would be encouraged for their sake and that of society to end their own lives willingly. But More's defense of euthanasia was a lot less than meets the eye. More meant the book to be largely fanciful and basically entertaining. In the final analysis, More was a thoroughly orthodox Catholic who persecuted heretics remorselessly and thus was a highly unlikely candidate to espouse heterodox views, information Catholics have used to try to defeat euthanasia advocates. See Sir Thomas More, "Utopia," in Zucker, ed., *The Right to Die Debate*, 228. See also Larson and Amundsen, *A Different Death*, 143, 145–46.

13. Gruman, "An Historical Introduction to Ideas about Voluntary Euthanasia," 87–138, quote on 90.

14. Minois, *History of Suicide*, 181–83.

15. American statutory laws derived from English common law, which held suicide to be a crime because it deprived the king of "property" in the form of one of his subjects. In the new republic, such royalist legal reasoning no longer applied.

16. Larson and Amundsen, *A Different Death*, 157. See also Friedman, "Suicide, Euthanasia, and the Law," 681–89; Crocker, "The Discussion of Suicide in the Eighteenth Century," 47–72. In 1902, the Texas Court of Criminal Appeals ruled that assisted suicide was legal in that state. This groundbreaking decision overturned the murder conviction of a Texas physician who had supplied his mistress with the gun she used to commit suicide. The suicide had taken place while the physician, his wife, his mistress, and another woman were discussing their sexual transgressions. Still, the court of appeals ruled that there was no crime if the victim was aware of the danger and desired self-destruction. Since Texas, like so many other states, had no law against suicide, it could not be a crime to aid and abet persons determined to kill themselves. Six years later, the Texas Court of Criminal Appeals similarly reversed the murder conviction of a ranch hand who provided his girlfriend with carbolic acid so she could kill herself. As in the 1902 ruling, the court conceded that the suicide had occurred under shady circumstances, but relying on a theory of rugged frontier individualism, it argued that the suicide knew perfectly well what she was doing. In other words, the court neglected to distinguish between rational suicides and those committed in a state of mental or emotional disorder. The Texas law that suicide was an entirely private act was not changed until 1973. Engelhardt, Erde, and Moskop, "Euthanasia in Texas: A Little Known Experiment," 30–31.

17. Pappas, "Recent Historical Perspectives Regarding Medical Euthanasia and Physician Assisted Suicide," 386–93, quote on 387; Fye, "Active Euthanasia," 494.

18. Lewis O. Saum, "Death in the Popular Mind of Pre-Civil War America," in Stannard, ed., *Death in America*, 30–48. For an insightful description of medical care

of the dying in Victorian England, resembling conditions in America, see Jalland, *Death in the Victorian Family*, 81–86.

19. For Paris medicine, see Erwin H. Ackerknecht, *Medicine at the Paris Hospital, 1794–1848* (Baltimore: The Johns Hopkins University Press, 1967); Dora B. Weiner, *The Citizen-Patient in Revolutionary and Imperial Paris* (Baltimore: Johns Hopkins University Press, 1993).

20. "The Euthanasia," *Medical Surgical Reporter* 29 (1873): 122–23.

21. Robinson, ed., "A Symposium on Euthanasia," 134–55, 154–55.

22. One exception to this trend among Anglo-American doctors was the eminent physician William Osler, who in 1905 endorsed chloroforming men sixty years of age or over to death, with or without their consent. I thank Michael Bliss for drawing this fact to my attention. See Michael Bliss, *William Osler, A Life in Medicine* (Toronto: University of Toronto Press, 1999), 323–28. See also Glick, *The Right to Die*, 13.

23. Starr, *The Social Transformation of American Medicine*, 145–46. See also Rosenberg, *The Care of Strangers*, 142–65.

24. For the transition from the "modern" to the "postmodern" patient, see Shorter, *Bedside Manners*, especially 107–39, 211–40.

25. Emanuel, "The History of Euthanasia Debates in the United States and Britain," 793–802, quote on 796.

26. A case in point was the groundbreaking essay, titled "Euthanasia," by Samuel D. Williams, a nonphysician member of the Birmingham Speculative Club in England. Williams recommended the use of chloroform to kill incurable and pain-ridden patients if they so desired. Excerpts from Williams's essay were reproduced in the American *The Popular Science Monthly* and demonstrate, among other things, how the debate over active euthanasia has not changed much since the late nineteenth century. Claiming nature "certainly knows nothing" about the human theory of the sacredness of life, he proceeded to justify a legal right to die on the basis of what use individuals make of their lives. When life is a burden to patients and they "can no longer be of use to others," then they are entitled to seek "a quick and painless death." Williams added that in "existing medical practice" doctors frequently administered drugs that relieved pain but shortened a patient's life. Reaction to Williams included warnings that legalizing active euthanasia would lead to abuses, such as the murder of invalids and infants, while putting pressure on the sick and the dying to avail themselves of euthanasia laws. "Euthanasia," *The Popular Science Monthly* 3 (1873): 90–96.

27. Abraham Jacobi, "Euthanasia," *Medical Review of Reviews* 18 (1912): 362–63, quote on 363.

28. Editorial, "The Moral Side of Euthanasia," *The Journal of the American Medical Association* 5 (1885): 382–83.

29. James Reed, "Doctors, Birth Control, and Social Values, 1830–1970," in Vogel and Rosenberg, eds., *The Therapeutic Revolution*, 109–33, quote on 112. See also James Reed, *From Private Vice to Public Virtue*. Reed's thesis that medical attitudes

toward contraception were primarily conditioned by the social values they shared with other Americans, rather than the state of contraceptive technology, is similar to this book's argument that the views of euthanasia advocates historically have been conditioned more by values and ideology than the changes in medical technology.

30. For accounts that stress the "schizophrenic composition" of Progressivism, see Graham, *The Great Campaigns*, 156; Wiebe, *The Search for Order, 1877–1920*; Rothman, *Conscience and Convenience*; Dewey, *Individualism, Old and New*, 36. For a penetrating analysis of these tensions in Progressive thought, see McClay, *The Masterless*, 148–52, 170–87.

31. Russett, *Darwin in America*, 133–35.

32. Conkin, *When All the Gods Trembled*, vii.

33. John Dewey, "The Influence of Darwin on Philosophy," in Appleman, ed., *Darwin: A Norton Critical Edition*, 305.

34. Hofstadter, *Social Darwinism in American Thought*, 86–87.

35. Among late-nineteenth-century American naturalists there is little evidence that exposure to Darwinism caused them to leave their respective churches. Numbers, *Darwinism Comes to America*, especially 40–43. Numbers questions the thesis of James Moore, who argued that evolution triggered "spiritual crises" in the lives of Anglo-Americans who had to contend with it. Moore, *The Post-Darwinian Controversies*, 109.

36. Ruse, *The Darwinian Revolution*, 70–74.

37. Numbers, *Darwinism Comes to America*, 33, 44. See also Darwin, *Origin*, 458.

38. He did remark near the end of the book that thanks to his theory "[l]ight will be thrown on the origin of man and his history." Darwin, *Origin*, 458.

39. Charles Darwin, *The Descent of Man and Selection in Relation to Sex*, 2 vols. (New York: D. Appleton, 1871), 2: 369.

40. Conkin, *When All the Gods Trembled*, 40, 43.

41. Ruse, *The Darwinian Revolution*, 247. See also Degler, *In Search of Human Nature*, 9.

42. Russett, *Darwin in America*, 214.

43. Ingersoll may have fulminated against Christianity, but he still subscribed to the Golden Rule, most of the Beatitudes, and the Sermon on the Mount. Wakefield, ed., *The Letters of Robert G. Ingersoll*, 702.

44. *The Complete Works of Robert Ingersoll*, 12 vols. (New York: C. P. Farrell, 1920), 2: 356–57, 8: 225, 11: 567–68. Quoted in John Rickards Betts, "Darwinism, Evolution, and American Catholic Thought, 1860–1900," *Catholic Historical Review* 45 (1959): 161–85, 171.

45. The "Agnostic and the Positivist," according to Ingersoll, "have the same end in view—both believe in living for this world." So admiring was Ingersoll of Comte that on his first trip to Europe in 1875 he visited the cemetery of Père-Lachaise in Paris to see Comte's tomb. Wakefield, ed., *The Letters of Robert G. Ingersoll*, 309n, 310, 525, 526, 642. For samples of Comte's thought, see Gertrud Lenzer,

ed., *Auguste Comte: The Essential Writings* (Chicago: University of Chicago Press, 1975).

46. For the impact of Comte's positivism on American liberal thought, see Harp, *Positivist Republic*, esp. xv–xvi, 213–16.

47. Wakefield, ed., *The Letters of Robert G. Ingersoll*, 3–66.

48. Wakefield, ed., *The Letters of Robert G. Ingersoll*, 698–704.

49. Hillel Levine, "Introduction" to Adler, *An Ethical Philosophy of Life Presented in Its Main Outlines*, 3k–4k.

50. *Chicago Tribune*, 6 August 1891, 1. Cited in Kuepper, "Euthanasia in America," 31–32.

51. Adler, *An Ethical Philosophy*, 179–81. His italics.

52. Edward S. Morse, "Address," *Proceedings of the American Association for the Advancement of Science* 36 (1887): 1–43, quote on 2. Cited in Numbers, *Darwinism Comes to America*, 38.

53. Darwin, *Descent of Man*, 1: 205–6, 212–13, 216. See also Hawkins, *Social Darwinism in European and American Thought, 1860–1945*, 35–38; Claeys, "The 'Survival of the Fittest' and the Origins of Social Darwinism," 223–40, quote on 237; Greene, "Darwin as a Social Evolutionist," 1–27. Saying that Darwin was a Social Darwinist is not the same as saying, however, that there was a single political message to derive from Darwinism.

54. For the links between the eugenics and euthanasia movements in England, see Ian Dowbiggin, "C. Killick Millard and the Euthanasia Movement in Great Britain, 1930–1955," *Journal of Contemporary History* 36 (2001): 59–85.

55. Francis Galton, *Inquiries into Human Faculty and Its Development* (London: J. M. Dent and Sons, 1883), 24. Quoted in Paul, *Controlling Human Heredity: 1865 to the Present*, 3.

56. See Stepan, *"The Hour of Eugenics"*; Broberg and Roll-Hansen, eds., *Eugenics and the Welfare State*. One example of this phenomenon was the membership list swapping of the Euthanasia Society of America and Birthright, Inc., a group that in its early years lobbied for eugenic sterilization laws. See Minutes of the Meeting of the [Birthright] Executive Committee, 23 November 1943, SWHA, SWD 15, Box 1, folder 7; Mrs. Myron Goldstein to Mrs. Robert Edwards, 10 May 1950, PFC, Box C-1.

57. Mehler, "A History of the American Eugenics Society, 1921–1940."

58. Dowbiggin, *Keeping America Sane*, 191–231.

59. Haller, *Eugenics*, 137. See also Pickens, *Eugenics and the Progressives*; Ludmerer, *Genetics and American Society*; Kevles, *In the Name of Eugenics*; Reilly, *The Surgical Solution*; Larson, *Sex, Race, and Science*; Rafter, *Creating Born Criminals*.

60. Pernick, "Eugenics and Public Health in American History," 1767–72.

61. Galton himself was notoriously anticlerical, castigating the Catholic Church for its defense of celibacy and even conducting experiments to try to prove that praying was a waste of time. Kevles, *In the Name of Eugenics*, 11, 68.

62. Wiggam, *New Decalogue of Science*, 22, 279.

63. Frank H. Hankins, "Irrationality of Birth Control," in Sanger, ed., *The Sixth International Neo-Malthusian and Birth Control Conference*, 192–93. Or, as another eugenicist proclaimed in 1928, the human race's "Duty to the Immortal Germ Plasm" translated into a new secular "religion." Alfred Scott Warthin, "A Biologic Philosophy or Religion," National Conference on Race Betterment, *Proceedings* 3 (1928): 86–90. Cited in Pernick, *The Black Stork*, 99.

64. G. Stanley Hall, *Life and Confessions of a Psychologist* (New York: Appleton, 1923). 357. Cited in Zenderland, "Biblical Biology," 511–25, 518. I wish to thank Ian Nicholson for drawing this source to my attention. Zenderland argues that there was not as much antagonism between Christianity and eugenics in America as some scholars originally believed. However, by focusing on reformist Protestant eugenicists and ignoring Roman Catholic opposition to eugenics, she has skewed her evidence.

65. After studying one such "degenerate" family, numbering 1,200 members over five generations, Dugdale concluded that they cost government over $1.3 million. Dugdale, *"The Jukes,"* 167.

66. Reilly, *The Surgical Solution*, 13–18.

67. Elks, "The 'Lethal Chamber,' " 201–7. See also Hollander, "Euthanasia and Mental Retardation," 53–61; Heifetz, "From Munchausen to Cassandra," 67–69.

68. Hollander, "Euthanasia and Mental Retardation," 57.

69. Sigmund Engel, *The Elements of Child-Protection*, trans. Eden Paul (New York: Macmillan, 1912), 257–58. Quoted in Pernick, *The Black Stork*, 23.

70. Pernick, *The Black Stork*, 23–24.

71. Kuepper, "Euthanasia in America," 36–38; Emanuel, "The History of Euthanasia Debates in the United States and Britain," 796.

72. Patterson, *America in the Twentieth Century*, 1–71.

73. Rosenberg, *The Care of Strangers*, 310–36.

74. Starr, *The Social Transformation of American Medicine*, 79–197; Porter, *The Greatest Benefit to Mankind*, 397–427.

75. Wiebe, *The Search for Order*, 134.

76. Graham, *The Great Campaigns*, 1, 2, 16–17, 155.

77. Arthur S. Link and Richard L. McCormick, *Progressivism* (Arlington Heights, Ill.: Davidson, 1983), 6–8.

78. Notable Progressives who aided the eugenics movement included President Theodore Roosevelt, Wisconsin governor Robert La Folette, Supreme Court justice Oliver Wendell Holmes, and New Jersey's governor (and later U.S. president) Woodrow Wilson. For the argument that eugenics was a Progressive reform movement, see Vecoli, "Sterilization: A Progressive Measure?" 190–202; Haller, *Eugenics*, 5; Pickens, *Eugenics and the Progressives*; Kevles, *In the Name of Eugenics*, 101; Larson, "Belated Progress," 44–64; Larson, *Sex, Race, and Science*, 30–31, 79–81, 88–89, 115–16, 131–39; Dowbiggin, *Keeping America Sane*, 124–31.

79. William J. Robinson, *Eugenics, Marriage, and Birth Control*, 2d ed. (New York: Critic and Guide, 1922), 74–76. Cited in Kevles, *In the Name of Eugenics*, 93–94.

For more on Robinson, see Gordon, *Woman's Body, Woman's Right*, 173–78; Pernick, *The Black Stork*, 27, 33, 69, 79, 82, 89, 93, 160, 166.

80. Robinson, "Euthanasia," 85–90. Cited in Kuepper, "Euthanasia in America," 38–39.

81. Robinson, ed., "A Symposium on Euthanasia," 134–55. Debs emphasized safeguards intended to prevent any abuses, but he did condone euthanasia for a "doomed sufferer" who had reached the "stage of mental irresponsibility." In that case, "those responsible for him" could petition for his death. Similarly, he argued that human life was "sacred, but only to the extent that it contributes to the joy and happiness of the one possessing it, *and to those about him*" (151–52; my emphasis).

82. As early as 1868 Haeckel had suggested killing impaired newborns. Ernst Haeckel, *The History of Creation*, vol. 1 (New York: D. Appleton, 1868), 170–71. Cited in Pernick, *The Black Stork*, p. 22. For Haeckel's defense of abortion, infanticide, and the mercy killing of the mentally ill, see Weikart, "Darwinism and Death."

83. Jack London to Ralph Kasper, June 1914, *Letters from Jack London*, ed. King Hendricks and Irving Shepherd (New York: Odyssey Press, 1965), 145. Quoted by Russett, *Darwin in America*, 176.

84. For London's Darwinist philosophy, see Russett, *Darwin in America*, 175–82.

85. Robinson, ed., "Symposium on Euthanasia," 152.

86. Ross's sympathy for birth control was colored by mainly eugenic motives. For Ross and the Wisconsin eugenics movement, see Vecoli, "Sterilization: A Progressive Measure?" 190–202. See also Haller, *Eugenics*, 92, 134, 147, 153, 167.

87. Patterson, *America in the Twentieth Century*, 11–31, 55–56, 171–72.

88. The advantage of positivist knowledge as a kind of "social religion" was that it simultaneously allowed someone to differ with orthodox Christian teaching yet retain religion's ability to buttress social solidarity. As the historian Gillis Harp has written, "Comtists could indulge themselves in the quasi-religious duty to doubt, while still providing for the emotional needs of individuals and preserving the moral 'cement' that they believed held society together." Harp, *Positivist Republic*, 17. See also Ross, *The Origins of American Social Science*, 233.

89. This point has been made most forcefully by Ezekiel Emanuel. See Emanuel, "The History of Euthanasia Debates in the United States and Britain," 793–802.

90. The prewar years were marked by mounting worry that the nation faced a "severe suicide crisis" over a seeming epidemic of suicide. Frederick L. Hoffman, the chief statistician for the Prudential Insurance Company, was the main source for the belief that suicide was on the rise. Kuepper, "Euthanasia in America," 25–29. Bolstering interest in voluntary death for the chronically ill were Hoffman's data that the incidence of cancer was increasing in early-twentieth-century America. What also emerged from Hoffman's data was the conclusion that more

and more Americans were escaping death from infectious diseases and surviving until middle and old age, when cancer most often struck. See Patterson, *The Dread Disease*, 79–82. American psychiatrists had been warning about an "epidemic" of suicide since the middle of the nineteenth century. See Kushner, "American Psychiatry and the Cause of Suicide, 1844–1917," 36–57.

91. Editorial, "Euthanasia," *British Medical Journal* 1 (1906): 638–39.

92. Speaking of the Bollinger baby, Haiselden declared: "Defectives are prolific. It would reproduce its kind." *Washington Post*, 17 November 1915. Cited in Pernick, *The Black Stork*, 207n. The theory that the mentally retarded were alarmingly fertile began to go out of fashion in serious medical circles by the early 1920s, when H. H. Goddard, an early defender of the theory, rejected it entirely. See Dowbiggin, *Keeping America Sane*, 101–2.

93. Pernick, *The Black Stork*, 49, 50, 60; Kuepper, "Euthanasia in America," 70.

94. Kuepper, "Euthanasia in America," 69–70.

95. Pernick, *The Black Stork*, 94.

96. Ibid., 41.

97. Ibid., 171.

98. Ibid., 14–15.

99. Madison Grant, *The Passing of the Great Race* (New York: Scribner's, 1916), 45, 47. Cited in Pernick, *The Black Stork*, 56.

100. Pernick, *The Black Stork*, 81–85. See also Kuepper, "Euthanasia in America," 62–63. In 1917 Irving Fisher changed his mind yet again about Haiselden's eugenic euthanasia, when he said that "eugenics does not require the old Spartan practice of infanticide." Irving Fisher and Eugene Lyman Fisk, *How To Live*, 12th ed. (New York: Funk and Wagnalls, 1917), 294. Cited in Pernick, *The Black Stork*, 160.

101. *Philadelphia Inquirer*, 18 November 1915, 7. Cited in Kuepper, "Euthanasia in America," 72.

102. Pernick, *The Black Stork*, 59.

103. "The Defective Baby," *New Republic* 5 (1915): 85–86.

104. Helen Keller, "Physicians' Juries for Defective Babies," *New Republic* 5 (1915): 43–44.

105. *New Orleans Morning Star*, 20 November 1915. Cited by Pernick, *The Black Stork*, 77.

106. John P. Carroll, "The Moral Side of the Bollinger Baby Case," *American Ecclesiastical Review* 54 (1916): 315–20, quote on 320.

107. Headline, *New World*, 26 November 1916, 1. Cited in Pernick, *The Black Stork*, 34.

108. *Medical Review of Reviews* 22 (1916): 123. Cited in Pernick, *The Black Stork*, 35.

109. "The Morality of Using Chloroform to Deaden Pain," *American Ecclesiastical Review* 20 (1899): 201–4; Cornelius O'Leary, "Euthanasia," *Catholic World* 62 (1896): 579–87, 584–85. See also Pope Pius XII, "The Prolongation of Life," in Zucker, ed., *The Right to Die Debate*, 62–63. For criticism of the "double-effect"

principle, see Williams, *The Sanctity of Life and the Criminal Law*, 322; Humphry and Clement, *Freedom to Die*, 190–93.

110. *Chicago Tribune*, 20 November 1915, 8, quoting *Baltimore Catholic Review*, 19 November 1915. Cited in Pernick, *The Black Stork*, 86.

111. See Hugh Cabot to Clarence C. Little, 9 November 1939, PFC, Box C-1. See also Pernick, *The Black Stork*, 30.

112. Pernick, *The Black Stork*, 160; Kuepper, "Euthanasia in America," 46–47. See also Hofstadter, *The Age of Reform: From Bryan to F.D.R.*, 302–3, 316.

Chapter 2

1. George H. Gallup, *The Gallup Poll: Public Opinion, 1935–1971*, 3 vols. (New York: Random House, 1972), vol. 1, 151.

2. Charles Francis Potter, *The Preacher and I: An Autobiography*, 363, 367.

3. "Mercy Killings," *Fortune* 16, (1937): 106.

4. "The Right to Kill," *Time*, 25 November 1935, 39–40. Kuepper, "Euthanasia in America," 120.

5. Kuepper, "Euthanasia in America," 95–96.

6. Carl Sandburg, *The People, Yes* (New York: Harcourt, Brace and World, 1936), 14–15. See also *New York Times*, 15 March 1932.

7. "Viewpoints," *Readers' Digest*, October 1935, 74; Charlotte Perkins Gilman, "The Right to Die–I," *The Forum* 94 (1935): 297–300. See also *New York Times*, 20 August 1935, 44.

8. "Viewpoints," *Readers Digest*, October 1935: 74. Gilman and Blatch, besides seeking the vote for women, also endorsed birth control. Catt declined to sponsor Margaret Sanger's American Birth Control League, founded in 1921, but her disagreement with Sanger had less to do with birth control than Sanger's claim that birth control alone held the key to the emancipation of women. See Gordon, *Woman's Body, Woman's Right*, 237–38.

9. Sherwood Anderson, "Dinner in Thessaly," *The Forum* 95, (1936): 40–41; Abraham Wolbarst, "The Right to Die," *The Forum* 94 (1935): 330–32. See also Abraham Wolbarst, "Syphilitic Heredity," *Eugenical News* 16 (1931): 112–13.

10. Degler, *In Search of Human Nature*, 59–104.

11. Reilly, *The Surgical Solution*, 45, 84, 88. See also Larson, *Sex, Race, and Science*.

12. The British physician A. F. Tredgold was a leader in this enterprise, inching his way toward a recommendation of euthanasia for the mentally retarded in the editions of his textbook between 1908 and 1952. See A. F. Tredgold, *A Textbook on Mental Deficiency* (New York: William Wood, 1908, 1915, 1920, 1922, 1929, 1937, 1947). See also Elks, "The 'Lethal Chamber,' " 201–7.

13. "Death for Insane and Incurable Urged by Illinois Homeopaths," *New York Times*, 9 May 1931, 4. This decision by the Illinois Homeopathic Medical Society was largely the idea of William A. Guild, a Chicago physician. See his "Euthanasia," *Journal of the American Institute of Homeopathy* 27 (1934): 82–83. William Partlow,

a leading southern psychiatrist, warned in the midst of his unsuccessful 1936 campaign to secure a sterilization law for Alabama that, if eugenic measures were not undertaken, "euthanasia may become a necessity." His sentiment was echoed by a Georgia psychiatrist in 1937 who predicted that if the country did not sterilize its "human rubbish," it would have to resort to euthanasia. Partlow never spoke for anything more than a small minority of American psychiatrists, but his words confirmed that eugenics and euthanasia continued to be linked in the minds of some Americans as late as the outbreak of World War II. That eugenics was gradually losing its status as a credible science hardly seemed to matter to people like Partlow. Larson, *Sex, Race, and Science,* 52, 146–47, 149, 154, 232 n.20.

14. Earnest Hooton, "The Future Quality of the American People," *The Churchman* 154 (1940): 11–12. See also Kuepper, "Euthanasia in America," 99–100.

15. William G. Lennox, "Should They Live? Certain Economic Aspects of Medicine," *The American Scholar* 7 (1938): 454–66. See also W. L. Funkhouser, "Human Rubbish," *Journal of the Medical Association of Georgia* 26 (1937): 197–99; Landman, *Human Sterilization,* 12. The Rockefeller Institute's Nobel Prize–winning scientist Alexis Carrel said criminals, psychotics, and incurably ill individuals should be gassed. See "The Right to Kill," *Time,* 18 November 1935, 53.

16. In 1938 Potter wrote that there appeared to be a "great popular interest in euthanasia in this country at this time. It would seem from the great numbers of clippings which daily come to [the ESA] office that America has suddenly become euthanasia-conscious." Potter to H. H. Greenwood, 11 February 1938, PFC, Box C-4.

17. Potter, *The Preacher and I,* 362.

18. See Kuepper, "Euthanasia in America," 109–10.

19. They were, in the words of one historian, "fighting evangelicals." Conkin, *When All the Gods Trembled,* 56.

20. Conkin, following William R. Hutchison, argues that the modernists of the 1920s were "a subclass of Protestant or evangelical liberalism." See Hutchison, *The Modernist Impulse in American Protestantism,* 257–87.

21. Peter J. Bowler, "Darwinism and Modernism: Genetics, Paleontology, and the Challenge to Progressionism, 1880–1930," in Ross, ed., *Modernist Impulses in the Human Sciences,* 236–54, quote on 244. For an account of the "crisis of modernity" and its implications for the history of the American Catholic Church, see Morris, *American Catholic,* 155–58.

22. Cited in Dorothy Ross, "Modernist Social Science in the Land of the New/Old," in Ross, ed., *Modernist Impulses in the Human Sciences,* 171–89.

23. Barnes, *The Twilight of Christianity,* 433–34, 453.

24. Fosdick, *Christianity and Progress,* 179, 186–87. Others were not as sanguine about science's capacity to help America navigate the coming years. In the 1920s, leading thinkers such as Walter Lippman and Joseph Wood Krutch worried about the damage the new sciences inflicted on orthodox religion. To Lippmann "the

acids of modernity" were destroying the old moral guidelines, but he was not as optimistic as Barnes or Fosdick about science's ability to replace the old conventions with a new morality that could guarantee freedom, maintain law and order, and preserve social solidarity. Krutch was even gloomier. In his *The Modern Temper* (1929), he stressed the destructive power of science and the way it demolished everything from romantic love to tragic drama. Modern human beings stood naked before a dismal future. Thus, Krutch and Lippman, despite their pessimism, agreed with Barnes and Fosdick that the coming of science meant America would never be the same again. See Conkin, *When All the Gods Trembled*, 158–68.

25. The best account of the Scopes trial is Larson, *Summer for the Gods*. For a similar treatment of the Dayton trial and its aftermath, which disposes of many of the myths surrounding fundamentalist interpretations of evolution and Bryan's performance on the stand, see Numbers, *Darwinism Comes to America*, 76–91.

26. Numbers, *Darwinism Comes to America*, 88.

27. Larson, *Summer for the Gods*, 117.

28. H. L. Mencken, "The Monkey Trial: A Reporter's Account," in Tomkins, ed., *D-Days at Dayton*, 40.

29. As historian Edward J. Larson observed, "[a]ll other courtroom prayers were directed exclusively to the Christian God." Larson, *Summer for the Gods*, 117.

30. For Potter's account of the founding of the First Humanist Society, see Potter, *The Preacher and I*, 356–98. See also Charles Potter, *Humanism: A New Religion* (New York: Simon and Schuster, 1930). By 1937 the First Humanist Society and its branch organizations overseas numbered about 15,000 members. See Charles Potter, "Unbelievers of Right and Left Wings," *Literary Digest* 123 (1937): 27–28.

31. Miller, *American Protestantism and Social Issues*, 167, 242–43, 312, 321–22, 324. The Unitarian journal *Christian Register* was more leftist than most Unitarian publications or groups, and repeatedly praised Stalin's Soviet Union in the 1930s as true to the teachings of Jesus Christ and the greatest experiment in all history (85).

32. David B. Parke, "A Wave at Crest," in Conrad Wright, ed., *A Stream of Light*, (Boston: Unitarian Universalist Association, 1975), 111. Cited in Robinson, *The Unitarians and the Universalists*, 143.

33. Charles Francis Potter, "A Message to America," broadcast in the "World of Religion Program," 25 June 1933 by the National Broadcasting Company. Http: // www.infidels.org / library / historical / charles_potter / message_to_america. html.

34. Potter, *The Preacher and I*, 377–78.

35. Perry Miller, "Individualism and the New England Tradition," in John Crowell and Stanford J. Searl, eds., *The Responsibility of Mind in a Civilization of Machines*, (Amherst: University of Massachusetts Press, 1979), 42. Cited in Robinson, *The Unitarians and the Universalists*, 154.

36. "Dr. Potter Backs 'Mercy-Killings,' " *New York Times*, 3 February 1936, 13. See also Charles Francis Potter, "Euthanasia: An Important Social Measure" and "The Formation of the Euthanasia Society of America," PFC, Box C-4.

37. Charles Francis Potter, "Mercy Deaths You Don't Hear About, or, Secret Euthanasia," c. 1939; "Mercy Deaths We Don't Hear About, or, Bootleg Euthanasia," c. 1938, PFC, Box C-4.

38. Elks, "The 'Lethal Chamber,' " 201–7, quote on 201.

39. Charles Francis Potter, "Euthanasia: Is Mercy-Killing Justified?" and "Mercy Deaths You Don't Hear About, or, Secret Euthanasia," PFC, Box C-4.

40. Potter, *Creative Personality*, 197–99.

41. "Dr. Inez Philbrick, 70, Fights for the First 'Mercy-Killing' Law," *The Milwaukee Journal Green Sheet*, 17 February 1937, ICP, Scrapbook.

42. Inez C. Philbrick letter to the editor, *Dayton Daily News*, 4 September 1947, ICP, Ms. 1058, Scrapbook. See also letter to the editor of an unidentified newspaper, n.d., Scrapbook.

43. "Safety and Food Value Paramount in Milk," *Dayton Daily News*, 3 July 1938, ICP, Scrapbook.

44. Philbrick's feminism was rooted in the suffrage movement. In 1920 the National American Woman Suffrage Association officially recognized her as a "Pioneer" of the cause, awarding her a Distinguished Service Certificate for her contributions to the campaign to win women the vote. Carrie Chapman Cott to Philbrick, 12 March 1920, ICP, Ms. 1058, folder 2.

45. Inez C. Philbrick, "Women: Let Us Be Loyal to Women," *Medical Women's Journal*, February 1929, ICP, Ms. 1058, folder 3.

46. Inez C. Philbrick, "Further Reflections on Euthanasia," n.d., ICP, Ms 1058, Scrapbook. See also Philbrick to C. Killick Millard, 6 March 1937, CMAC/SA/VES/Box 3/A.19.

47. Philbrick relied heavily on the advice of State Senator and attorney John H. Comstock. The thirty-two-year-old Comstock agreed to help draft the bill not only because he believed in euthanasia; he also warmly admired Philbrick, who had delivered him as a baby.

48. Nebraska Legislature, 52nd Session, "Legislative Bill No. 135."

49. Inez C. Philbrick to Charles Francis Potter, 20 December 1937, PFC, Box B-1.

50. Despite some support from a few local clergymen and the lay public, state politicians tended to ignore the Philbrick/Comstock bill. After public hearings before the legislature's Committee on Public Health and Miscellaneous Subjects, a motion by the only physician in the legislature that the bill be indefinitely postponed was carried without dissent, ending Philbrick's Nebraska initiative.

51. Inez Celia Philbrick, "Radio Talk on Euthanasia," n.d., PFC, Box B-1.

52. Thomas M. Peery, "The New and Old Diseases: A Study of Mortality Trends in the United States, 1900–1969," *American Journal of Clinical Pathology* 63 (1975), 458. Cited in Majorie B. Zucker, ed., *The Right to Die: A Documentary History*, 29–30.

53. "Mercy Bill Filed in Nebraska," *New York Times*, 14 February 1937; "Mercy Death Bill Killed in Committee," *Lincoln Star*, 24 February 1937.

54. She hoped that her brother-in-law, the editor of the Dayton *Daily News*, as well as H. H. Goddard, the expert on mental retardation who had expressed guarded interest in euthanasia, might be able to help her achieve what she could not in the Cornhusker state. For Philbrick's plans, see Bessie Moore to Charles Francis Potter, 15 December 1938, PFC, Box B-1. Moore was Philbrick's Ohio attorney. Goddard, befitting his skepticism about the diagnosis of feeblemindedness, could not agree with Philbrick on euthanasia for the mentally retarded and generally was doubtful about the wisdom of trying to introduce euthanasia bills. Charles Francis Potter to Philbrick, 26 October 1938, ICP, Ms. 1058, folder 2; H. H. Goddard to C. C. Little, 6 May 1941, PFC, Box C-1.

55. For Mitchell's statement of "the facts of my family history as my mother told them to me," n.d., see PFC, Box E-1. Mitchell's reference to a "monster birth bill" can be found in an undated letter to an unknown correspondent, PFC, Box E-1.

56. See "Notes Made of Mr. Sidney G. Soon's Statement to Mr. Tompkins and Mrs. Jones, Monday, October 19th in Mr. Mitchell's Presence," PFC, Box E-1.

57. Dowbiggin, " 'A Prey on Normal People,' " 59–85

58. For the notion that euthanasia and eugenics were "based on the same fundamental idea as to man's place in the universal scheme," see Dr. Harry Roberts, "Doctors and the 'Right to Die,' " *Nottingham Guardian*, 29 December 1931.

59. C. Killick Millard to Potter, 31 December 1936, ICP, Ms. 1058, Scrapbook.

60. See Potter to Millard, 23 December 1937, CMAC/SA/VES/Box 3/A.19. See also "Sanction Is Sought for 'Mercy Deaths,' " *New York Times*, 17 January 1938, 21; "Editorial," *New York World Telegram*, 25 January 1938.

61. Potter to Millard, 12 January 1939, CMAC/SA/VES/Box 3/A.19.

62. Ann Mitchell to Mrs. Robert E. Simon, 5 July 1942, PFC, Box E-1. For Potter's account of these events, see *The Preacher and I: An Autobiography* (New York: Crown, 1951), 396–99.

63. See Potter's letter of resignation to the ESA Board of Directors, 20 December 1938. See also his letter to Millard, 9 February 1939, PFC, Box C-4. An example of his assertion that he had founded the ESA is his letter to Robert Sherrod, 16 May 1962, PFC, Box C-4. For the feminist credentials of ESA women, see Garrett, "The Last Civil Right?" 31. For similar developments within the birth control movement, see Gordon, *Woman's Body, Woman's Right*, 255; McCann, *Birth Control Politics in the United States, 1916–1945*, 197–98.

64. Valery Garrett came up with this percentage by comparing the names of NSLE board members with members and officers of various eugenics groups or authors of pro-eugenic essays from *Eugenical News* (1916–1945). Garrett, "The Last Civil Right?" 24n.

65. Wiggam to Potter, n.d., PFC, Box C-4. In 1923 Wiggam maintained that "killing off the weaklings" was in fact "anti-eugenical" or "dysgenic," although he did not

explain why—nor did he say whether he opposed involuntary active euthanasia for terminally ill persons for noneugenic purposes. See Wiggam, *The New Decalogue of Science*, 100.

66. See Mitchell to C. Killick Millard, 31 March, 27 September, 17 December 1939, 2 April, 7 May 1940, 20 October 1941, 14 June, 4 July, 18 August 1942, CMAC/SA/VES/A.19–20/Box 3.

67. Charles Nixdorff to C. Killick Millard, 8 May 1939, PFC, Box C-3.

68. See Charles Potter, "The Formation of the Euthanasia Society of America," PFC, Box C-4; see also clipping from the *Austin (Minnesota) Herald*, 7 February 1938; PFC, Box C-1.

69. "Dr. Goodsell Dead; Taught at Columbia," *New York Times*, 1 June 1962, 28. See Robert E. Engel, "Willystine Goodsell: Feminist and Reconstructionist Educator," *Vitae Scholasticae* 3 (1984): 355–78. For Goodsell's eugenic views, see Willystine Goodsell, "The New Eugenics in Education," *The Social Frontier* 4 (1938): 113–17.

70. See Abraham Myerson et al., *Eugenical Sterilization: A Reorientation of the Problem* (New York: Macmillan, 1936). See also Myerson, "A Critique of Proposed 'Ideal' Sterilization Legislation," *Archives of Neurology and Psychiatry* 33 (1935): 453–66; "Abstract: The Sterilization Question," *Psychiatric Quarterly* 10 (1936): 158–64. Potter actually thought that "in some quarters the suggestion of euthanasia for incurable idiots meets with readier acceptance than the suggestion of voluntary euthanasia for sane sufferers." Potter to Millard, 14 March 1938, CMAC/SA/VES/Box 3/A.19.

71. Minutes of the 30 March 1938 meeting of the board of directors of the National Society for the Legalization of Euthanasia, PFC, Box C-3. According to Potter, euthanasia for "incurable idiots" was the ESA's "ultimate aim." Potter to Millard, 1 April 1938, CMAC/SA/VES/Box 3/A.19.

72. See "Proposed Bill to Legalize Euthanasia," published by the Euthanasia Society of America, Inc., n.d.; also "Mercy Death Law Proposed in State," *New York Times*, 27 January 1939, 21; "Mercy Death Law Ready for Albany," *New York Times*, 14 February 1939, 2.

73. "Indifference Is Evil, Rev. Gannon Tells Catholics," *Pelham (N.Y.) Sun*, 26 May 1939. See also "Mercy-Killing Scored," *New York Times*, 27 February 1938, 4; "Euthanasia Opposed by Catholic Group," *New York Times*, 19 February 1939, 5. For her complaint that "the legislature of New York State [was] almost entirely controlled by Catholics," see Mrs. R. L. Mitchell to C. Killick Millard, 31 May 1939, CMAC/SA/VES/Box 3/A.19. See also Mrs. R. (Gertrude Ann) Edwards to Millard, 10 February 1945, CMAC/SA/VES/Box 3/A.20.

74. "Dr. S. E. Goldstein, Family Authority," *New York Times*, 21 March 1955, 25. See also "Rabbi Asks in Church for More Family Life," *New York Times*, 21 September 1925; "Calls on Churches to Unite for Peace," *New York Times*, 25 January 1932; "Urges Men Accept Minor Role in Home," *New York Times*, 21 October 1932; "Finds Race Aided by Birth Control," *New York Times*, 20 January 1933; "Peace Fight Urged by Drive on Voters," *New York Times*, 21 May 1936.

75. Minutes of the 3 May 1938 meeting of the NSLE board of directors, PFC, Box C-1.

76. "Mercy Death Law Ready for Albany," *New York Times*, 14 February 1939, 2. See also Kennedy's letter to the editor of the *New York Times*, 22 February 1939, 20; "Doctor's Defence of Euthanasia," *Daily Telegraph* (London), 15 February 1939.

77. Foster Kennedy, "The Problem of Social Control of the Congenital Defective," *American Journal of Psychiatry* 99 (1942): 1–4.

78. For Kennedy's statement that his views were "entirely personal and in no way to be construed as the policy of the E.S.A.," see his letter to the editor, *New York Times*, 22 February 1939. See also Charles Nixdorff to Millard, 21 February 1939, CMAC/SA/VES/Box 3/A.19.

79. Eleanor Dwight Jones to Mrs. Caspar Whitney, 10 March 1939, PFC, Box C-2.

80. Second Annual Meeting of the Euthanasia Society of America, PFC, Box C-4.

81. "Report of the Work of Dr. Inez Celia Philbrick," c. 1942, CMAC/SA/VES/Box 3/A.20.

Chapter 3

1. Friedlander, *The Origins of Nazi Genocide*, xii. See also Götz et al., *Cleansing the Fatherland: Nazi Medicine and Racial Hygiene*, 92; Burleigh, *Death and Deliverance*, 220–66; Weindling, *Health, Race, and German Politics between National Unification and Nazism, 1870–1945*, 548, 551. For a recent account of the German nurses' complicity in Nazi euthanasia, see Benedict and Kuhla, "Nurses' Participation in the Euthanasia Programs of Nazi Germany," 246–64. Leo Alexander, a Boston psychiatrist who served on the staff of the Office of the Chief Counsel for War Crimes at Nuremburg, compiled the first postwar report on Nazi euthanasia and was also the first to argue that history showed Nazi euthanasia "started from small beginnings." Alexander, "Medical Science Under Dictatorship," 39–47, quote on 44. See also Marrus, "The Nuremberg Doctors' Trial in Historical Context," 106–23.

2. Michael Burleigh, in his seminal *Death and Deliverance* (1994), contends that Nazi medicine's mass murder of vulnerable social groups should not be called euthanasia, and therefore he places the word in quotation marks. As this book makes clear, I disagree. Because there is no way of knowing precisely where present-day right to die reform will lead, and because the Nazis themselves referred to their practices as euthanasia, there is no reason to stop using the term to describe what happened between 1939 and 1945. See Burleigh, *Death and Deliverance*.

3. Burleigh, *Death and Deliverance*, 238.

4. Racial hygiene was a term coined by the German physician Alfred Ploetz (1860–1940).

5. Weindling, *Health, Race, and German Politics*, 115–18. See also Sheila Faith Weiss,

Race, Hygiene, and National Efficiency: The Eugenics of Wilhelm Schallmayer (Berkeley and Los Angeles: University of California Press) 1987.

6. For the impact of Darwinism on German attitudes toward euthanasia, eugenics, and abortion, see Weikart, "Darwinism and Death: Devaluing Human Life in Germany, 1859–1918." See also Hans-Walter Schmühl, *Rassenhygiene, Nationalsozialismus, Euthanasie: Von der Verhutung zur Vernichtung 'lebensunwerten Lebens', 1890–1945* (Göttingen: Vandenhoek und Ruprecht, 1987).

7. Burleigh, *Death and Deliverance*, 12–14. I am indebted to Professor Richard Weikart for his thoughts on the ties between Darwinism and the "de-valuing of life" in German history.

8. Robert J. Lifton, *The Nazi Doctors: Medical Killing and the Psychology of Genocide* (New York: Basic Books, 1986), 48.

9. Binding borrowed the phrase "negative value of life" from author Adolf Jost, who had coined it in 1895. Weindling, *Health, Race, and German Politics*, 394.

10. Karl Binding and Alfred Hoche, "Permitting the Destruction of Unworthy Life: Its Extent and Form," trans. Walter E. Wright, Patrick G. Derr, and Robert Salomon, *Issues in Law and Medicine* 8 (1992): 231–65, 231–55.

11. Weindling, *Health, Race, and German Politics*, 394–95.

12. Binding and Hoche, "Permitting the Destruction of Unworthy Life," 255–65. Hoche's emphasis.

13. Michael Burleigh, "Psychiatry, German Society, and the Nazi 'Euthanasia' Programme," *Social History of Medicine* 7 (1994): 213–28.

14. Burleigh, *Death and Deliverance*, 183–219. By January 1945 *Ich klage an* had been seen by over 15 million people, 275,000 seeing it in Munich alone (216).

15. Burleigh, *Death and Deliverance*, 45; Weindling, *Health, Race and German Politics*, 545–46.

16. Kater, *Doctors Under Hitler*, 54–88.

17. The pretext for the beginning of Nazi euthanasia had occurred in 1938, when Hitler was sent a request from a family for the killing of their crippled child in a Leipzig clinic. In fact, Hitler and various medical officials in the Third Reich had already decided by then to begin an extermination program of congenitally handicapped newborns and children.

18. Michael R. Marrus, "Resisting the Slippery Slope," *University of Toronto Bulletin* 13 March 2000, 20. See also Marrus, "The Nuremburg Doctors' Trial in Historical Context," 106–23. For similar reflections on "playing the Nazi card" and seeing implications of Nazi medicine where few exist, see Proctor, *The Nazi War on Cancer*, 270–71.

19. Michael Straight, "Germany Executes Her Unfit,' " *New Republic* 5 (May 1941): 627–28; William L. Shirer, "Mercy Deaths in Germany," *Reader's Digest,* July 1941, 55–58. See also William L. Shirer, *Berlin Diary: The Journal of a Foreign Correspondent, 1934–1941* (New York: Knopf, 1941), 512, 569–75.

20. C. Killick Millard to Ann Mitchell, 17 February 1940, PFC, Box C-3.

21. Mitchell to Millard, 27 September, 17 December 1939, 2 April, 7 May 1940, 20

October 1941, 4 July, 18 August 1942, CMAC/SA/VES/Box 3/A.20. Millard was decidedly less enthusiastic than Mitchell about Nazi euthanasia and observed that it would "not raise much sympathy anywhere." Millard to Mitchell, 10 September 1941, PFC, Box C-3.

22. For American eugenicists and their sympathy toward Nazi eugenic sterilization, see Kühl, *The Nazi Connection.*

23. ESA Board minutes, 7 April 1943, PFC, Box C-3. Tompkins, an 1897 graduate of Vassar, helped found the League of Women Voters. She was also a longtime American Birth Control League board member. See her obituary, *New York Times*, 1 March 1947. See also Frank Hinman, "Euthanasia," *Journal of Nervous and Mental Diseases* 99 (1944): 640, 643, for a review of ESA literature and its temporary decision to stress the desirability of voluntary euthanasia rather than a "right to kill."

24. "Debate-Town Hall Cracker-Barrel Forum: Should Voluntary Mercy Death (Euthanasia) Be Legalized?" 16 February 1943, PFC, Box C-4. Potter probably realized his mistake in invoking the impending return of the veterans as a justification for euthanasia, because in 1947 he debated the same question on CBS Radio and made no mention of any veterans' demands to be euthanized. See "Script for Discussion of 'Should Voluntary Euthanasia Be Legalized?' " PFC, C-4; Potter to Eleanor Dwight Jones, n.d. (but probably 1943), PFC, Box C-4. The addition in 1943 of William G. Lennox to the ESA's advisory council was yet another indication of the heterodox opinions tolerated in the organization. This was the same Lennox who had written in 1938 that involuntary sterilization might have been used to solve Germany's "Jewish problem." In 1950 Lennox was still calling for the mercy killing of "children with undeveloped or misformed brains" as a way of opening up space in "our hopelessly clogged institutions." William G. Lennox, "The Moral Issue," c. 1950, PFC, Box C-1.

25. Kuepper, "Euthanasia in America," 114. See also "Mrs. F. Robertson Jones Dead: Birth Control Movement Leader," *New York Times*, 31 July 1965, 21.

26. Sanger was a member of the ESA advisory board from 1942 until her death in 1965, a fact overlooked by all her biographers. Although her interest in euthanasia could be partly traced to her deteriorating health in the 1950s and 1960s, Sanger's affiliation with the ESA dated back to her days in the birth control and eugenic movements. She and Jones were alike precisely because they believed that "the same people who think courageously enough to plan birth should also accept the right to plan death," as Sanger put it. Eleanor Dwight Jones to Mrs. [?] Groves, 15 October, n.d., PFC, Box C-3. For Jones quoting Sanger again, see Eleanor Dwight Jones to Mr. [?] Churchill, 24 April 1951, PFC, Box C-1. See also "Eleanor Dwight Jones," PFC, Box C-1; Margaret Sanger to Pauline Taylor, 2 February 1959, PFC, Box C-4. For Jones's involvement in the birth control movement and her relations with Margaret Sanger, see Chesler, *Woman of Valor*, 238–42; McCann, *Birth Control Politics in the United States, 1916–1945*, 177–78, 180–81. Chesler's efforts to draw fundamental distinctions between Sanger and

Jones ignore the many similarities in their overall mentalities, similarities that show up in their respective interests in euthanasia. In addition, Chesler, like all biographers of Sanger, fails entirely to mention Sanger's affiliation with the ESA, which stretched over more than two decades.

27. See Jones to the Coronet Round Table, 17 November 1944, PFC, Box C-1.

28. Dickinson influenced the work of sexologist Alfred C. Kinsey, introducing Kinsey to "Mr. X," the polymorphously erotic man whom Kinsey studied closely and on whom Kinsey based many of his theories about human sexual behavior. Jones, *Alfred C. Kinsey,* 291, 503–8.

29. Reed, *From Private Vice to Public Virtue,* 161–62.

30. For Dickinson's contributions to the birth control movement, see Reed, *From Private Vice to Public Virtue,* 143–93. For Dickinson's vision of a "broad program to improve the quality of life," see ibid., 185. See also McCann, *Birth Control Politics,* 79–81, 82–91; Chesler, *Woman of Valor,* 269–88, 372–75.

31. Birthright, Inc., an organization that, like the ESA, has gone through several name changes since World War II, is now called EngenderHealth.

32. As Birthright's president told Dickinson in 1948,

> if the half wits and morons could be talked into sterilization after the birth of a few children, instead of making no attempt to limit their numbers at all, we could at least be getting somewhere. I and several of my friends are doing them quite often on these women on a strictly voluntary basis and it is not hard to talk most of them into it during their pregnancies. They do not want to be bothered with a lot of children and when it is explained to them are only too happy to have it done. We need to educate the doctors to educate the patients.

H. Curtis Wood to Robert Latou Dickinson, 22 November 1948, SWHA, SWD 15, Box 2, folder 15. For the early history of Birthright, Inc., see William Ray Vanessendelft, "A History of the Association for Voluntary Sterilization, 1935–1964" (Ph.D. diss., University of Minnesota, 1978).

33. Margaret Sanger was a sponsor of Birthright in the 1950s and 1960s and a vocal advocate of the theory that American states should offer incentives to the mentally handicapped to undergo sterilization. Sanger's involvement in Birthright and its later incarnation as the Human Betterment Association of America, like her involvement in the ESA, has been largely overlooked by her biographers. For Sanger and Birthright, see "Copy," "Address by Margaret Sanger," and "Sterilization: A Modern Medical Program for Human Health and Welfare," SWHA, SWD 15.1, Box 18, Sanger Folder. These documents prove that between the 1920s and her death in 1965 Sanger never gave up her eugenic hopes for birth control. For a different interpretation of Sanger's eugenicism, see Chesler, *Woman of Valor,* 417.

34. Radio broadcast by Dickinson, 16 December 1946, on CBS Radio's "In My Opinion" show, RLD, Box 3, folder 27.

35. "1,000 Doctors Urge 'Mercy Death' Law," *New York Times,* 15 December 1947, 30.

36. For example, see "No Compromise," *New England Journal of Medicine* 242 (19 January 1950): 107–8.

37. *Los Angeles Times*, 10 March 1950, Pt. 1, 11. Cited in Kuepper, "Euthanasia in America," 229.

38. John Blum, *From the Morgenthau Diaries: Years of War, 1941–1945* (Boston: Houghton Mifflin, 1967), 72. Cited in Starr, *The Social Transformation of American Medicine*, 279. See also ibid., 273.

39. Philip R. Reilly, *The Surgical Solution: A History of Involuntary Sterilization in the United States* (Baltimore: Johns Hopkins University Press, 1991) 144; Blanshard, *American Freedom and Catholic Power*, 145; Lader, *Politics, Power, and the Church*, 72–74. For an example of Catholic pressure on birth control clinic physicians, see Sister Anna Rita to Dr. Armand DeRosa, 8 January 1942, SWHA, SWD 15, Box 1, folder 4; Henry J. Olson of the Los Angeles Planned Parenthood Center to the editor of the *New York Herald Tribune*, 4 January 1960, clipping in SWHA, SWD 15, Box 4, folder 37.

40. Bert Voorhees to the ESA, 11 February 1948, PFC, Box C-3.

41. At least one doctor threatened to sue the ESA, although the official Catholic newspaper of the Archdiocese reported that his card recording his assent to the petition could be found in the ESA files. See Floyd Anderson, "Who Signed for Euthanasia?" *America* 96 (1957): 573.

42. Stephen H. Curtis to Dickinson, 30 January 1948, PFC, Box C-3.

43. For example, see A. Kent MacDougall, "Euthanasia: Murder or Mercy?" *The Humanist* 18 (1958): 38–47, 44. In fact, age-adjusted rates of cancer mortality rose very slowly in the 1940s and 1950s. Patterson, *The Dread Disease*, 159.

44. William S. McCann to Eleanor Dwight Jones, 28 January 1952, PFC, Box C-1.

45. Patterson, *The Dread Disease*, 125, 137–39, 149–51, 191. See also L. Lander, *Defective Medicine: Risk, Anger, and the Malpractice Crisis* (New York: Farrar, Straus, and Giroux, 1978), 41. Cited in John C. Burnham, "American Medicine's Golden Age: What Happened to It?" *Science* 215 (1982): 1474–79, quote on 1477.

46. "The Law of God," *Time*, 16 January, 1950, 20; "Not Since Scopes?" 13 March 1950, 43. Potter, the veteran of the Darrow-Bryan showdown in 1925, predicted that the Sander trial would be "another Scopes trial." *New York Post*, 18 January 1950. In ten days of court sessions, the press corps filed 1,600,000 words. Fannie Hurst was one reporter in Manchester, filing stories for the Boston *American*. As a member of the ESA, Hurst was hardly an impartial observer.

47. Millard's own exploitation of the Sander case in the English press can be found in CMAC, SA/VES/Box 6/B.7. For Jones on the Sander trial, see "U.S. Society Will Seek Law Permitting 'Mercy-Killings,' " *New York Herald Tribune*, 4 January 1950. See also "Ministers Back 'Mercy Killer'," *New York Times*, 25 January 1950, 19; "The Mercy Killing," *New Republic* 122 (1950): 6.

48. Editorial, "A House in Order," *New England Journal of Medicine* 242 (1950): 842–43.

49. The VESC was also able to attract prominent Yale University figures, such as

Roland H. Bainton, the noted historian of religion, and the eugenicist psychologist Robert Mearns Yerkes. Yale's Sterling Law School professor Wesley A. Sturges fully endorsed the VESC's stand on elective euthanasia but declined to join the organization, pleading other commitments.

50. "Proposed Bill: A Suggested Solution to the Problem of Relief for Those Incurable Sufferers Who Desire Euthanasia," the Voluntary Euthanasia Society of Connecticut, PFC, Box C-3.

51. Isabel Tarrant to Eleanor Dwight Jones, 3 April 1950, PFC, Box C-3.

52. See Eleanor Dwight Jones's comments in the *ESA Bulletin*, January 1950, 3.

53. Yale Kamisar, "Some Non-Religious Views Against Proposed 'Mercy-Killing' Legislation," *Minnesota Law Review* 42 (1958): 969–1042, 1019–20. As a New York State senator and assemblyman charged, Potter's defense of Sander was the same thing as calling John Dillinger a "saint." Potter's weak defense was to say that at least Sander had "focused attention on the fact that the law is far behind public sentiment," itself a highly questionable statement. "Immediate Release: From Dr. Charles Francis Potter," 11 January 1950, PFC, Box C-4.

54. Robert L. Dickinson, "Statement To Be Signed by Members of This Committee," 13 January 1950, PFC, C-3. See also A. L. Wolbarst to Anne Gertrude Edwards, 4 October 1949, PFC, Box B-5. For Millard's protests that the VELS sought only a "right to die," not a "right to kill," see his letter to the editor of the *Glasgow Herald*, 8 December 1950, CMAC/SA/VES/Box 6, B.7.

55. Morris, *American Catholic*, 195.

56. Ibid., 184, 223.

57. For Dougherty, see Morris, *American Catholic*, 165–95. For Spellman, see Cooney, *The American Pope*.

58. Harold A. Fey, "Can Catholicism Win America?" *Christian Century* (8-part series), 61–62 (29 November 1944–17 January 1945). Often home to anti-Catholic, Protestant opinions, the *Christian Century* did publish Edgar N. Jackson's "Is Euthanasia Christian?" 67 (8 March 1950): 300–301. The author, while not condemning euthanasia outright, argued that "in a society that is increasingly preoccupied not with individuals but with economic and social goals," it was important for all Christians to think long and hard about the practice before trying to legalize it. See Morris, *American Catholic*, 224–25; Allitt, *Catholic Intellectuals and Conservative Politics in America, 1950–1985*, 16; Dolan, *The American Catholic Experience*, 384–417.

59. For Coughlin, see Morris, *American Catholic*, 145–49.

60. For the tensions between American liberals and Catholics in the post–World War II years, see McGreevy, "Thinking on One's Own," 97–131.

61. That led to the ironic situation in which the Roman Catholic Church became the most stalwart defender of U.S. laws against contraception, such as the Massachusetts and Connecticut statutes originally passed by Protestant politicians in the nineteenth century, and outlawing the dissemination and use of contraceptives.

62. Kinsey's data have not stood the test of time well. For confirmation, see Kinsey's revealing biography by James H. Jones, *Alfred C. Kinsey: A Public/Private Life.*

63. Burnham, "The Influence of Psychoanalysis upon American Culture," in Burnham, *Paths into American Culture*, 96–112. See also Burnham's "The Progressive Era Revolution in American Attitudes Toward Sex," ibid., 150–66.

64. Allitt, *Catholic Intellectuals and Conservative Politics*, 163–203. See also Reed, *From Private Vice to Public Virtue*, 67–139, 281–316.

65. Patterson, *America in the Twentieth Century: A History*, 357–58.

66. "Make It Legal?" *Time*, 18 November 1948, 70.

67. See "Legalization of Voluntary Euthanasia: Statement on the Ethical Aspect by Fifty Religious Leaders of N.Y. State" and "Petition to the Legislature of the State of New York," PFC, Box C-3. See also "Protests of Euthanasia Petition Held 'Irrelevant,'" *Buffalo Courier-Express*, 30 January 1949.

68. Conkin, *When All the Gods Trembled*, 121.

69. Union Theological Seminary had once been Presbyterian, but in 1893 it disaffiliated and became a hotbed of religious liberalism, steering young minds such as Fosdick's away from systematic theology and toward a version of Christianity that emphasized its ethical dimensions and the intense personal experience of faith. Fosdick, *The Living of These Days*, 19–22, 49, 76, 279.

70. Conkin, *When All the Gods Trembled*, 121–28.

71. Fosdick to Eleanor Dwight Jones, 10 December 1943, PFC, Box C-3.

72. To Fosdick, "[i]ndiscriminate human spawning serves no useful purpose." Fosdick quoted by H. Curtis Wood, "The Case for Voluntary Sterilization," *The Humanist* 29 (1969): 3–4. For Fosdick's involvement in Birthright, see SWHA, SWD 15, Box 2, folder 12, especially Fosdick to Marian Olden, 14 June 1945. For Fosdick's comments on the ESA and euthanasia, see Fosdick, *The Living of These Days*, 284–85.

73. Eleanor Dwight Jones to Harry S. Meserve, 23 February 1949, PFC, Box C-3; Jones to Bert Voorhees, 14 February 1948, PFC, Box C-3. Birthright's Marian Olden concurred, applauding Charles Potter's 1947 radio broadcast, "The Case for Voluntary Euthanasia," for "expos[ing] the methods of that church which acts as an obstacle to progress in every form." Marian Olden to Charles Potter, 2 February 1947, PFC, Box C-4.

74. "Dr. Coffin Is Dead: Headed Seminary," *New York Times*, 26 November 1954, 29; Henry Sloane Coffin, "American Freedom and Catholic Power," *Christianity and Crisis*, 2 May 1949, 49–51, 49. Quoted in John T. McGreevy, "Thinking on One's Own," 127–28.

75. Eleanor Dwight Jones to Guy Emery Shipler, 18 February 1947, PFC, Box C-3.

76. "Euthanasia: Protestant and Jewish Clergy Ask Humane Ethics," *The Churchman*, 15 January 1949, 19; "Protestants United Open Their Campaign" and "The Mission of the POAU," *The Churchman*, 15 February 1949, 10–11; George A. Coe, "Euthanasia: The Issue's Core," *The Churchman*, 15 February 1951, 12–13 (Coe, at one time professor of education at Teachers' College, Columbia University,

taught at Union Theological Seminary); Earnest A. Hooten, "The Future Quality of the American People," *The Churchman*, 1 September 1940: 11–12.

77. Blanshard, *American Freedom and Catholic Power*, 152, 154; Blanshard to Irene Headley Armes, 4 October 1951, SWHA, SW 15.1, Box 22, Blanshard Folder. As historian Philip Reilly has written, "[b]y the 1940s, the Catholic Church had embarked on a sustained drive against eugenic sterilization laws." Reilly, *The Surgical Solution*, 120.

78. Blanshard, *American Freedom and Catholic Power*, 125–27. For the review of Blanshard's book, see Euthanasia Society of America *Bulletin*, August–September 1949, 4.

79. Horace M. Kallen, *The Liberal Spirit: Essays on the Problems of Freedom in the Modern World* (New York: Cornell University Press, 1948), 220. Quoted in Gottfried, *After Liberalism: Mass Democracy in the Managerial State*, 61. So enamored was Kallen with statist solutions that, in 1927, he applauded Benito Mussolini's version of social planning in fascist Italy. For Kallen's admiration—albeit temporary—of Mussolini, see John P. Diggins, *Mussolini and Fascism: The View from America* (Princeton: Princeton University Press, 1972). For a trenchant critique of Kallen's theory of liberalism, see Gottfried, *After Liberalism*, 66, 75, 84–86, 101–2, 107. As Gottfried writes, Kallen's apology for Mussolini does not make him a fascist, but it does indicate that social planners like Kallen rather carelessly were looking for models that might be applied to American society (157, n. 53).

80. Kallen, "An Ethic of Freedom," 1164–69, quote on 1169.

81. Horace Kallen to Alice M. Proskauer, 15 February, 17 October 1957, HK, Correspondence, Box 25, folder 20.

82. Blanshard, *American Freedom and Catholic Power*, 7. Blanshard's *The Nation* articles were reprinted as *The Roman Catholic Church in Medicine, Sex, and Education* (New York: The Nation, 1948). See also Harry Benjamin, "A Humane Necessity," *The Nation* 170 (1950): 79–80. As Stephen Kuepper notes, Benjamin was one of the few physicians to write in favor of active euthanasia between 1945 and the 1960s. Kuepper, "Euthanasia in America, 1890–1960," 285, n. 53.

83. See "Euthanasia Is the Answer," *The Truth Seeker* 76 (November 1949): 165. The journal defended Hermann Sander's actions. See "God, Pain, and Euthanasia," *The Truth Seeker* 77 (February 1950): 26–27. Its position on euthanasia has been fairly consistent up to the present day, publishing the writings of Jack Kevorkian and Derek Humphry. See issue 5, *The Truth Seeker* 121 (1994).

84. Cooney, *The American Pope*, 177–85.

85. " 'Mercy Killing' Scored," *New York Times*, 27 February 1938, 4; "Euthanasia Opposed by Catholic Group," *New York Times*, 19 February 1939, 5. See also Kuepper, "Euthanasia in America," 131.

86. "Vatican Condemns 'State' Euthanasia," *New York Times*, 6 December 1940, 25; "Pope Places Limits on the Right to Kill," *New York Times*, 14 November 1944, 9.

87. "Mercy Bill Scored by Church Jurist," *New York Times*, 9 December 1946, 28; "Dr. Potter Replies to Euthanasia Foe," *New York Times*, 16 December 1946, 35. For

other incidents in the late 1940s when Potter defended the ESA against attacks from Catholic organizations, see Potter's (unpublished) letter to the editor of the *New York Times*, 17 December 1947, PFC, Box C-4. Potter was replying to an allegation by the New York State commander of the Catholic War Veterans that the ESA proposal to legalize voluntary euthanasia was a "product of Hitler's Nazi Germany" and "spawned by an atheistic totalitarian regime."

88. "Mercy-Killing Plea Hit," *New York Times*, 7 January 1949, 15; " 'Mercy Killings,' Called Murder," *New York Times*, 10 January 1949, 23; "Euthanasia Forbidden by the Bible," *News from the American Council of Christian Churches*, February 1949, PFC, Box C-1. See also "Euthanasia Critics Lauded by Cardinal," *New York Herald Tribune*, 7 May 1950; "Lauds Euthanasia Stand," *New York Times*, 7 May 1950; "Cardinal Lauds Medical Unit's Euthanasia Ban," *New World* (Chicago, Ill.), 26 May 1950.

89. " 'Mercy' Deaths Hit by Catholic Women," *New York Times*, 19 August 1947, 25.

90. "Medical Series Is On: In Lectures at Rockhurst, Priest Explains Catholic View," *Kansas City Times*, 15 September 1949; John Cogley (editor of *The Commonweal*) to Eleanor Dwight Jones, 1 February 1950, PFC, Box C-1; "The Sanctity of Life," *America* 101 (1959): 667.

91. For examples of warnings by Catholics as early as 1936 that the legalization of euthanasia would make America look like Nazi Germany, see *New York Times*, 6 January 1936, 12.

92. Shirley A. Patterson to the ESA, 27 September 1958, PFC, Box C-1.

93. "Let's Kill the Poor Beasts," *America* 80 (1949): 423–24. See also James Cardinal Gibbons, "The Moral Aspect of Suicide," *Century* 73 (1907): 401–7; "Mundelein Sees Church Menaced," *New York Times*, 6 January 1936, 12. As others insisted, there were sound nonreligious reasons why the "wedge" theory was correct. See Kamisar, "Some Non-Religious Views Against Proposed 'Mercy-Killing' Legislation."

94. "Murder or Mercy?" *Newsweek*, 3 February 1958, 56. Potter also told *Newsweek* that the ESA had 2,000 members, although a more accurate estimate would have been less than half that total.

95. "Murder or Mercy?" 56.

96. This is what the seventy-nine-year-old Harry Emerson Fosdick told *Newsweek* in 1958. See "Murder or Mercy?" 56.

97. George H. Gallup, *The Gallup Poll: Public Opinion, 1935–1971.* 3 vols. (New York: Random House, 1972), vol. 2, 887. See also Humphry and Wickett, *The Right to Die*, 38; Glick, *The Right to Die*, 57.

98. "World Medical Unit to Admit Doctors from Germany and Japan," *New York Times*, 18 October 1950, 22.

99. Eleanor Dwight Jones, no title, 10 October 1951, PFC, Box C-1.

100. Author's telephone interview with Donald W. McKinney, 21 December 1999.

101. MacDougall, "Euthanasia: Murder or Mercy?" 41.

102. Larson and Amundsen, *A Different Death*, 165.

Chapter 4

1. Death emerged as a dominant theme in music, film, poetry, and fiction. Kenneth L. Woodward, "How America Lives with Death," *Newsweek*, 6 April 1970, 81–88. See also Filene, *In the Arms of Others*, 49–50.

2. Pope Pius XII, "The Prolongation of Life: An Address of Pope Pius XII to an International Congress of Anesthesiologists," in Horan and Mall, eds., *Death, Dying, and Euthanasia*, 281–92. See also "The Pope's Views on Relief of Pain," *New York Herald Tribune*, 25 February 1957, 6; "Pope Grants Use of Pain Reliever," *New York Times*, 25 February 1957, 1.

3. Morris, *American Catholic*, 219–21. For Spellman's close friendship with Eugenio Pacelli (Pius XII), see Gannon, *The Cardinal Spellman Story*, 66ff, 81–89, 132ff, 153–75, 177–230, 283–94, 408–17; Cooney, *The American Pope*, 40, 41–42, 64–75, 111–19, 157–61, 183, 184, 198, 298–99.

4. For Spellman's attitudes toward sex, see Cooney, *The American Pope*, 109.

5. Fletcher, *Morals and Medicine*. See also Warren T. Reich, "The Word 'Bioethics': Its Birth and the Legacies of Those Who Shaped Its Meaning," *Kennedy Institute of Ethics Journal* 5 (1995): 319–36; Albert R. Jonsen, *A Short History of Medical Ethics* (New York: Oxford University Press, 1999); Robert Martensen, "The History of Bioethics: An Essay Review," *Journal of the History of Medicine and Allied Sciences* 56 (2001): 168–75. I wish to thank Professor Martensen for bringing these titles to my attention.

6. Joseph Fletcher, *Situation Ethics: The New Morality* (Philadelphia: Westminister Press, 1966).

7. According to Derek Humphry, Fletcher was a great help to him as a kind of "advisor" during Humphry's early years organizing the Hemlock Society in America. Author's telephone interview with Derek Humphry, 13 December 2001.

8. Joseph Fletcher, "The Patient's Right to Die," *Harper's Magazine* 221 (October 1960): 139–43, quote on 143.

9. Fletcher, *Morals and Medicine*, 174. His emphasis.

10. Joseph Fletcher, "Hospital Policy and Voluntary Sterilization: Is There an Infringement of Human Rights?" Speech at the HBAA annual meeting, 27 January 1959, New York City, SWHA, SWD 15, Box 4, folder 38.

11. *Contemporary Authors*, vol. 135, 156. But even those who disagreed vehemently with Fletcher admired his affable demeanor and respected his sincerity and candor. See Richard John Neuhaus, "All Too Human," *National Review* (2 December 1991): 45; "Dr. Joseph F. Fletcher, 86, Dies; Pioneer in Field of Medical Ethics," *New York Times*, 30 October 1991, D25.

12. Fletcher, *Morals and Medicine*, 170, 205, 209.

13. Degler, *In Search of Human Nature*, 185–211.

14. Holmes, *Life and Morals*, v. Holmes particularly praised educator John Dewey for his "hostility to 'antinaturalism' " and Dewey's call for a "moral science" that

needed to be divorced from theology and the doctrines of organized religion (viii, 5, 16).

15. Fletcher was the nephew of Irene Headley Armes, HBAA's executive director until her death in 1955. During the 1950s he had little to do formally with the HBAA, although he did tell the organization in 1956 to "count me in the company of your sympathizers. I only wish there was more I could do." Fletcher to Ruth Proskauer Smith, 11 February 1956, SWHA, SW15.1, Supplement, Box 15, Fletcher folder.

16. According to Fletcher, forcible sterilization was justified not only for eugenic and social purposes but also because the personal quality of life for children born to handicapped parents was so low. Fletcher, *Morals and Medicine*, 162–71. His emphasis.

17. Fletcher, *Morals and Medicine*, 174, 176. Elsewhere, Fletcher similarly dodged the issue of eugenic euthanasia, merely saying that simply because people endorsed voluntary euthanasia and "involuntary euthanasia for monstrosities at birth and mental defectives," it did not mean they logically had to support eugenic euthanasia. Joseph Fletcher, "Our Right to Die," *Theology Today* 8 (1951): 202–12.

18. Joseph Fletcher, "Ethics and Euthanasia," in Horan and Mall, eds., *Death, Dying, and Euthanasia*, 301. See also Linda Everett, "Right to Die Society Reveals Aims: To Kill Infants, Elderly," *New Federalist* (13 January 1989); Joseph Fletcher, "The Patient's Right to Die," *Harper's* 221 (1960): 140. Fletcher's book was open to another criticism. Alan Guttmacher, who would soon join Fletcher as an active member of the ESA, read Fletcher's manuscript and in 1953 said it was "a poor job and I am certain *no popular* [his] publisher will have a thing to do with it. It is verbose, poor style with too many defining parentheses. Furthermore his medical facts are curiously fallacious; I tried to correct many of them. I just feel the whole thing is hopeless." Alan Guttmacher note to Irene Headley Armes, 14 January 1953, SW15.i, supplement, Box 15, Fletcher folder.

19. Kallen, "An Ethic of Freedom" 1168, 1169. See also Horace Kallen to Mrs. Joseph M. Proskauer, 15 February 1957, HK, American Jewish Archives, Correspondence, Box 25, folder 20.

20. Paul Ramsey, "Freedom and Responsibility in Medical and Sex Ethics: A Protestant View," *New York University Law Review* 31 (1956): 1189–1204.

21. Claude R. Sowle, "How Should the Law Approach Mercy Killing?" 19 October 1959, PFC, Box C-1.

22. Williams, "Euthanasia and Abortion," 179.

23. Williams's book was based on his 1956 James S. Carpentier lectures at Columbia University. G. Williams, *The Sanctity of Life and the Criminal Law*, ix–x.

24. Williams, *The Sanctity of Life and the Criminal Law*, 346–50; Williams, "Euthanasia and Abortion," 181.

25. Kamisar, "Some Non-Religious Views Against Proposed 'Mercy-Killing' Legislation," 974. For Williams's answer to Kamisar, see his " 'Mercy-Killing' Legislation—A Rejoinder," in Horan and Mall, eds., *Death, Dying, and Euthanasia*, 480–91.

26. Kamisar, "Some Non-Religious Views Against Proposed 'Mercy-Killing' Legislation," 975, 1011. For Williams's response to Kamisar, see " 'Mercy-Killing' Legislation—A Rejoinder," *Minnesota Law Review* 43 (1958): 1–12.

27. Kamisar, "Some Non-Religious Views Against Proposed 'Mercy-Killing' Legislation," 976.

28. Alexander, "Medical Science Under Dictatorship," 44. See also Marrus, "The Nuremberg Doctors' Trial in Historical Context," 106–23.

29. Kamisar, "Some Non-Religious Views Against Proposed 'Mercy-Killing' Legislation," 976, 1032, 1038. His emphasis. He concluded (1031) by warning that

Miss Voluntary Euthanasia is not likely to be going it alone for very long. Many of her admirers, as I have endeavored to show in the preceding section, would be neither surprised nor distressed to see her joined by Miss Euthanatize the Congenital Idiots and Miss Euthanatize the Permanently Insane and Miss Euthanatize the Senile Dementia.

30. Joseph Fletcher, "Dysthanasia: The Problem of Prolonging Death," *Tufts Folio Medica* 8 (1962): 30–35.

31. Kuepper, "Euthanasia in America," 310.

32. In 1960, one subscriber asked, "Is the Society completely inactive?" Mrs. Robert Avery to the ESA, 16 March 1960, PFC, Box C-2. "For a year now I have been trying to get an answer—somehow from the Society," another lamented in 1967; "my letters were not returned so I know they must have been received, but never answered so I had made up my mind that [the ESA] had gone out of existence." Mrs. Walter S. Miller to the ESA, 24 November 1967; Robert W. Lawson to the ESA, 3 February 1969, PFC, Box C-2.

33. In the words of one supporter, across the country there was an "all too limited number of individuals who are thoughtful enough to be deeply aware and concerned about the principles involved in euthanasia. The trouble is due not to anything the Society has done or left undone, but to the apathy, indifference and irrational prejudices of the public." William J. Fielding to Pauline Taylor, 21 April 1964, PFC, Box C-4. As late as 1968 one member complained about the ESA's "snail's pace" and the "defeatist attitude of our supporters." Nancy Mamis to Mary Charlotte Peters, 28 February 1968, PFC, Box C-2.

34. On 13 February 1964, Heyde hanged himself in his cell. Burleigh, *Death and Deliverance*, 284.

35. Longtime member Frank Hankins admitted in 1964 that "the identification with Nazis is embarrassing to us." Frank Hankins to Pauline Taylor, 1 April 1964, PFC, Box C-4; Pauline Taylor to ESA Advisory Council Members, [?] March 1964, PFC, Box C-4. For more on Hankins, see Degler, *In Search of Human Nature*, 193–96.

36. Pauline Taylor to Mrs. Fermor S. Church, 4 March 1964, PFC, Box C-2.

37. Pauline Taylor to Charles Potter, 4 June 1959, PFC, Box C-2. The ESA's requests for tax-exempt status faced resistance from the IRS on the grounds that it was not a "social welfare" organization because it sought "the putting to death of human life by means of euthanasia [which] is contrary to all State law, and is

contravention of public policy." Sidney Rosoff to Pauline Taylor, 19 November 1962, PFC, Box C-2; Director, Tax Rulings Division, U.S. Treasury Department, Internal Revenue Service to the ESA, 9 November 1964, PFC, Box C-2.

38. Pauline Taylor to Dr. [?] Heiser, 18 April 1962, PFC, Box C-4. See also Walter Alvarez's form letter to other physicians (n.d., but probably late 1960s), encouraging the medical profession to enter into a "dialogue" with the ESA over the question of euthanasia. PFC, Box C-2.

39. He also had served as a consultant to the U.S. delegation when the United Nations Charter had been formulated in 1945. "John Paul Jones, Minister, Is Dead," *New York Times*, 6 March 1965, 34C.

40. Although McKinney knew something about the organization, it was only after a conversation with Roger Baldwin of the American Civil Liberties Union that he agreed to become a board member. Author's telephone interview with Donald W. McKinney, 21 December 1999; Minutes of Concern for Dying's board meeting, 28 October 1981, PFC, Box F-4.

41. Author's telephone interview with Donald W. McKinney, 21 December 1999.

42. Nancy Mamis to Johanna Graf, 1 February 1965; Kay Mali to Mrs. Walter N. Rothschild, 1 October 1965, PFC, Box C-2.

43. Author's interview with Ruth Proskauer Smith, 11 November 2000, New York City.

44. As she told *People* magazine in 1975, "death [has] followed sex as the last taboo." Christopher P. Andersen, "In Her Own Words," *People*, 17 March 1975, 43. See also "Katharine Strauss Mali, Headed Group Advocating 'Right to Die,' " *New York Times*, 26 June 1980.

45. Wertenbaker, *Death of a Man*. The book documents the last three months journalist and novelist Charles Wertenbaker and his wife Lael, then living in France, spent together as he died from inoperable liver cancer. See also Filene, *In the Arms of Others*, 48–49.

46. Euthanasia Society of America, Inc., "General Statement on the Purpose and Program of the Euthanasia Society of America"; Donald McKinney to Kay Mali, Florence Clothier, Ruth Proskauer Smith, 1 October 1965; Memo from Donald McKinney to Members of the ESA Board of Directors, 7 October 1965, PFC, Box D-1; Minutes of ESA Board meetings, 18 January, 28 September 1965, PFC, Box C-2.

47. Nancy Mamis to Johanna Graf, 1 February 1965, PFC, Box C-2.

48. Decades later, Derek Humphry and Mary Clement contended that "without the legacy of the 1960s," "what is now legal in Oregon [physician-assisted suicide] would probably still be second-degree manslaughter today." Humphry and Clement, *Freedom to Die*, 27.

49. For a version of this argument, see Emanuel, "The History of Euthanasia Debates in the United States and Britain," 793–802. However, I disagree with Emanuel's thesis that interest in euthanasia historically has been driven by the forces of Gilded Age and Reaganite "individualistic conservatism."

50. Critchlow, *Intended Consequences*, 156–57.

51. For insightful thoughts on this subject, see McClay, *The Masterless*, 235.

52. This applied especially to the expertise of "the best and the brightest," author David Halberstam's description of the liberals, intellectuals, and academics whose ideas shaped government policy in the early 1960s. Patterson, *America in the Twentieth Century*, 407.

53. Patterson, *America in the Twentieth Century*, 423–48; Patterson, *The Dread Disease*, 252.

54. Starr, *The Social Transformation of American Medicine*, 379.

55. Filene, *In the Arms of Others*, 68.

56. Rothman, *Strangers at the Bedside*, 64. The thalidomide tragedy caused a deluge of media articles on the subject in 1962, a number that is "equal to or exceeds those published in 1975 on the Karen Quinlan case." Glick, *The Right to Die*, 73.

57. Russell D. Wright, *Life and Death in the United States* (Jefferson, N.C.: McFarland and Co., 1997), 26–27. Cited in Valery Garrett, "The Last Civil Right?" 108.

58. Comments of Joseph Fletcher at the Third Euthanasia Conference, New York, N.Y., 5 December 1970. Cited in A. J. Rock Levinson, "An Overview of the Euthanasia Movement in the United States Today," prepared for the International Symposium on the Dying Human, Tel Aviv, Israel, 15–20 January 1978, 4.

59. Historian Peter Filene describes this as "the paradox of medical progress. . . . The more successful physicians became in curing disease and prolonging life, the more they were also held accountable for prolonging suffering." Filene, *In the Arms of Others*, 5.

60. *Life*, 11 August 1972, 38–39.

61. Lewis Thomas, "Dying as Failure," in "The Social Meaning of Death," Renee C. Fox, ed., *Annals of the American Academy of Political and Social Science* 447 (1980): 1–4. L. Lander, *Defective Medicine: Risk, Anger and the Malpractice Crisis* (New York: Farrar, Straus and Giroux, 1978), 41. Cited in Burnham, "American Medicine's Golden Age," 1477.

62. Toynbee quoted in Kenneth L. Woodward, "How America Lives with Death," *Newsweek*, 6 April 1970, 81.

63. Shorter, *Bedside Manners*, 211–40.

64. Starr, *The Social Transformation of American Medicine*, 335, 346–47.

65. Patterson, *The Dread Disease*, 233; Shorter, *Bedside Manners*, 216.

66. Starr, *The Transformation of American Medicine*, 391–92.

67. Filene, *In the Arms of Others*, 69–70.

68. McClay, *The Masterless*, 283–87, explores this topic with special lucidity.

69. For the considerable sympathy of nurses toward passive euthanasia and their actual performance of the practice, see Norman K. Brown et al., "How Do Nurses Feel About Euthanasia and Abortion?" *American Journal of Nursing* 7 (1971): 1413–16; Norman K. Brown and Donovan J. Thompson, "Non-Treatment of Fever in Extended-Care Facilities," *New England Journal of Medicine* 300 (1979): 1246–50. Cited in Filene, *In the Arms of Others*, 62, 238n.

70. See Jalland, *Death in the Victorian Family*, 98–104; Filene, *In the Arms of Others*, 134.

71. Anne Fadiman, "Death News: Requiem for the *Hemlock Quarterly*," *Harper's Magazine*, April 1994, 74; J. Holden, "Demographics, Attitudes, and Afterlife Beliefs of Right-to-Life and Right-to-Die Organization Members," *Journal of Social Psychology* 133 (1993): 521–27. A 1983 survey of early Hemlock Society membership found that 65 percent were women. Membership was overwhelmingly white and well educated, with most coming from Protestant backgrounds. Monica Surber et al., "Who Believes in Voluntary Euthanasia? A Survey of the Hemlock Society Membership," *Hemlock Quarterly* 12 (1983): 4–8. Cited in Garrett, "The Last Civil Right?" pp. 171–72.

72. Comments of Ruth Proskauer Smith at the annual SRD board meeting, 11 December 1989, PFC, uncatalogued.

73. Richard Bates, "It's Our Right to Pull the Plug," *Medical Economics*, 16 May 1977, FC, carton 1, folder 40.

74. Michel Vovelle, "Rediscovery of Death Since 1960," in Fox, ed., *The Annals of the American Academy of Political and Social Science* 447 (1980): 89–99.

75. Donald W. McKinney, *Whose Life Is It Anyway?* (Brooklyn: First Unitarian Church, n.d.), 1.

76. Peter Steinfels, "Introduction," in Steinfels and Veatch, eds., *Death Inside Out*, 1.

77. Lifton quoted in Woodward, "How America Lives With Death," 81.

78. Daniel Goleman, "We Are Breaking the Silence About Death," *Psychology Today* 10 (1976): 44. Suicides among the 15–24-year-old class rose 264 percent between 1950 and 1972. Over the same years, suicides for those aged 25–34 rose 152 percent. Jeanne Binstock, "Choosing to Die," *Futurist* 8 (1974): 68–71. Cited in Garrett, "The Last Civil Right?" 113.

79. Garrett, "The Last Civil Right?" 118.

80. *Death With Dignity: An Inquiry into Related Public Issues*, Proceedings Before the Special Committee on Aging, U.S. Senate, 92nd Congress, 2nd Session, 7–9 August 1972, Parts 1–3 (Washington, D.C.: Government Printing Office, 1972), Part 1, 1, Part 2, 68–69 (hereafter cited as *Death With Dignity*).

81. *Death With Dignity*, Part 2, 54–64.

82. "When Are You Really Dead?" *Newsweek*, 18 December 1967, 87.

83. Martin S. Pernick, "Brain Death in a Cultural Context: The Reconstruction of Death, 1967–1981," in Youngner, Arnold, and Schapiro, eds., *The Definition of Death*, 3–33; "Defining Death," *Time*, 10 March 1975, 76. See also Filene, *In the Arms of Others*, 56–59. Information on Beecher's friendship with Fletcher was obtained from historian Gary Belkin, personal communication, 24 January 2002.

84. Elisabeth Kübler-Ross, *On Death and Dying* (New York: Collier Books, 1969), 8, 16, 19; *Death With Dignity*, Part 1, 10–22, quote on 12. See also David Dempsey, *The Way We Die: An Investigation of Death and Dying in America Today* (New York: Macmillan, 1975), 14. One study that failed to verify Kübler-Ross's model was Richard Schulz and David Aderman, "Clinical Research and the Stages of Dying," *Omega* 5 (1974): 137–43.

85. Steinfels, "Introduction," 2, 3; Editorial, "Dying Is Worked to Death," *Journal of the American Medical Association* 229 (1974): 1909–10; Ronald J. Cohen, "Is Dying Being Worked to Death?" *American Journal of Psychiatry* 133 (1976): 575–77.

86. Steinfels, "Introduction," 2–4.

87. Filene, *In the Arms of Others*, 55.

88. Donald McKinney to the editor of the *New York Times*, 14 February 1966, PFC, Box D-1; Nancy Mamis to Barry Gray, 24 February 1966, PFC, Box C-2.

89. For reflections on how terminology about and attitudes toward death were "in flux" during the 1950s and 1960s, see Filene, *In the Arms of Others*, 9–10.

90. Donald McKinney to A-J Rock Levinson, 15 December 1976, PFC, Box D-1.

91. Kay Mali, "President's Report," EEC annual conference, 7 December 1974, PFC, Box D-1.

92. Nancy Mamis to Robert Kotlowitz, 24 February 1966, PFC, Box C-2.

93. Robert W. Lawson to J. Frank Schulman, 6 April 1970; J. Frank Schulman to Donald McKinney, 4 May 1970, PFC, Box D-1.

94. For the sullying of the word "eugenics" in the 1960s, see Kevles, *In the Name of Eugenics*, 251; Degler, *In Search of Human Nature*, 203–6.

95. Nancy Mamis, "Report on Planning Meeting of New Hampshire Committee on Population Problems, 29 July 1965," PFC, Box D-1. See also Nancy Mamis to Ralph Borsodi, 15 September 1965, PFC, Box C-2.

96. Elizabeth Halsey to Mrs. Harold Hays, 5 October 1971, PFC, Box C-2.

97. See *Euthanasia Society Bulletin* (June–July 1949). Cited in Garrett, "The Last Civil Right?" 128.

98. Luis Kutner, "Due Process of Euthanasia: The Living Will, a Proposal," *Indiana Law Journal* 44 (1969): 539–54. In 1967 Kutner (1908–1993), a cofounder of Amnesty International in London, discussed the idea of a living will at a meeting of the ESA.

99. Abigail van Buren, "Dear Abby," who would remain a stalwart friend of the euthanasia movement for the balance of the twentieth century, first advocated living wills in April 1973. In her columns she urged her readers to write to the EEC for a copy of the living will and enclose a financial contribution to cover the cost of reproducing and mailing the document. See "Dear Abby," "Some Thoughts on a 'Good Death,' " *Universal Press Syndicate*, 1 April 1973; reproduced in Zucker, ed., *The Right to Die Debate*, 75–76; A-J Rock Levinson, "An Overview of the Euthanasia Movement in the United States Today" (1978), PFC, Box F-4. Abby's April 1973 column led to a "crisis in the Euthanasia office," with staff and volunteers busily "sorting thousands of letters, extracting the money and answering the most urgent." So much cash and so many checks arrived that they had to be deposited several times a day in a nearby bank. Kay Mali to the EEC Board of Directors, 7 May 1973, FC, carton 1, folder 34.

100. Walter C. Alvarez, "Dear Doctor," n.d. (but a handwritten note claims it was the late 1960s), PFC, Box C-2. This was a form letter sent to doctors "who recognize the occasional need for euthanasia."

101. Sackett reconciled his Catholicism with his pro-euthanasia views by saying that he only wanted to allow people to die "the way God originally intended, before science has made it possible to prolong life." Walter Sackett to Olive Ruth Russell, 21 May 1969, NAC, MG31-K13, vol. 2, file 18. In 1976 Sackett was defeated for reelection by a younger challenger, an uncommon event in state politics, and it is likely that his reputation as a one-issue legislator had something to do with it. For more on Sackett, see Glick, *The Right to Die*, 104–9.

102. Arthur Levinsohn, "Voluntary Mercy Deaths: Socio-Legal Aspects of Euthanasia," *Journal of Forensic Medicine* 8 (1961), 68; Robert H. Williams, "Our Role in the Generation, Modification, and Termination of Life," *Archives of Internal Medicine* 124 (1969): 229–30. Cited in Filene, *In the Arms of Others*, 62, 238n.

103. To two physicians on staff, the infants had "acquired the right to die." For the "furious debate" within medicine because of these deaths, see Filene, *In the Arms of Others*, 114. See also "Deformed Infants Are Allowed to Die," *Washington Post*, 28 October 1973, B5; "The Hardest Choice," *Time*, 25 March 1974; Raymond S. Duff and A.G.M. Campbell, "Moral and Ethical Dilemmas in the Special Care Nursery," *New England Journal of Medicine* 289 (1973): 890–94; Rothman, *Strangers at the Bedside*, 194–204.

104. *Death With Dignity*, Part 1, 33. See also Walter W. Sackett, Jr., "I've Let Hundreds of Patients Die. Shouldn't You?" *Medical Economics* 50 (1973): 92–97; Russell, *Freedom to Die*, 189.

105. The state House of Representatives had passed his 1973 bill, only to have it die on the Senate calendar. Walter Sackett, "Death With Dignity" Report to the Florida House of Representatives, 7 August 1972, FC, carton 1, folder 34. "Death With Dignity," *Miami Herald*, 22 November 1970, 2C; " 'Death' Bill Put in Hopper Again," *Naples Daily News*, 13 January 1974. See also Kaplan, "Euthanasia Legislation: A Survey and a Model Act," 56.

106. Kaplan, "Euthanasia Legislation"; "Recent Euthanasia Legislative Activity in the U.S.A.," June 1974, PFC, Box D-1. The unsuccessful Montana initiative started because of the efforts of Joyce Franks, a housewife and mother of two children, who after watching her 85-year-old father die after breaking his hip, decided to lobby for support among state legislators for a euthanasia bill. Her second proposed bill was modeled closely after Sackett's, and permitted "passive euthanasia" even in cases when the patient had not consented beforehand. "Housewife Pleads for Right-to-Die Law," *Miami Herald*, 5 February 1972. Her lengthy correspondence with Olive Ruth Russell and Ruth Roettinger can be found in NAC, MG31-K13, vol. 2, file 18.

107. "Governor McCall's Views on the Death-With-Dignity Issue," Press release, 28 February 1972, NAC, MG31-K13, vol. 2, file 18. See also Russell, *Freedom to Die*, 193; Garrett, "The Last Civil Right?" 135–37.

108. Russell, *Freedom to Die* (Supplement to the 1st ed.), 396.

109. Neary and Brown, "The Veterans' Charter and Canadian Women Veterans of the Second World War," 249–77.

110. Olive Ruth Russell, "Women Tomorrow," address to University Women's Club, Dalhousie University, Halifax, Nova Scotia, 15 March 1944, NAC, MG31-K13, vol. 2, file 1. For more on Russell's feminism, see Ruth Swallow, "Olive Ruth Russell: A 20th Century Progressive" (master's thesis, University of Western Ontario, 1996), 133, 137n.

111. Olive Ruth Russell, "Freedom to Choose Death: A Discussion of Euthanasia," lecture given at the Chevy Chase Presbyterian Church, 20 May 1973, NAC, MG31-K13, vol. 2, file 16; *Freedom to Die*, 238–39. Russell's deep interest in the conditions of the hospitalized mentally retarded is evident from the many newspaper clippings on the topic in NAC, MG31-K13, vol. 3, file 28.

112. Olive Ruth Russell to Elizabeth Halsey and Kay Mali, 14 August 1972, NAC, MG31-K13, vol. 2, file 21. See also Judy Flander, "She Knows Meaning of Euthanasia: Psychologist Relates a Personal Story," *Washington Star*, 29 December 1975.

113. Russell, *Freedom to Die*, 19–22.

114. She became so disenchanted with its seeming conservatism that she eventually believed it had been infiltrated by people from the fledgling right-to-life movement. Olive Ruth Russell to Frances Graves, 21 September 1978, NAC, MG31-K13, vol. 2, file 18.

115. According to Ruth Roettinger, Russell was good friends with Fletcher, who encouraged her to translate her interest in the history of euthanasia into a book on the topic. Telephone interview with Ruth Roettinger, 25 May 2001. The foreword to *Freedom to Die* (3–4) was written by Helen Taussig (1898–1986), professor emeritus of pediatrics at the Johns Hopkins Medical School. Taussig joined the board of directors of the Society for the Right to Die in 1976. She had first gained notoriety in 1944 for devising with Dr. Alfred Blalock the "blue baby" operation, which saved the lives of thousands of children whose skin turned blue because of a lack of oxygen caused by birth defects of the heart. Later she helped to prevent the thalidomide disaster from spreading to the United States by publicizing the epidemic's cost in West Germany. "Dr. Helen Taussig, 87, Dies; Led in Baby Blue Operation," *New York Times*, 22 May 1986.

116. Russell, *Freedom to Die*, 90–93, 227.

117. Algernon Black, "Can Humanism Meet Man's Spiritual Need?" *The Humanist* 19 (1959): 195–206, quote on 200; Khoren Arisian, "Ethical Culture as a Contemporary Religious Humanism," *The Humanist* 35 (1975): 18–21.

118. ESA *Bulletin* 8 (1959): 1–4; Russell, *Freedom to Die*, 207.

119. This is no surprise, given that some who belonged to the AHA and Ethical Culture societies also belonged to the ESA. See Julius Kaunitz, "Legalizing Voluntary Euthanasia," *The Ethical Outlook* 43 (1957): 129–31; Jerome Nathanson, "The Right to Die," *The Humanist* 29 (1969): 25–30; Walter Alvarez, "Death With Dignity," *The Humanist* 31 (1971): 12–14. See also A. Kent MacDougall, "Euthanasia: Murder or Mercy?" *The Humanist* 12 (1958): 38–47. In 1997 the AHA filed an *amicus curiae* (friend of the court) brief with the U.S. Supreme

Court in favor of physician-assisted suicide. M. L. Tina Stevens, "What *Quinlan* Can Tell Kevorkian About the Right to Die," *The Humanist* (March/April 1997): 10–14.

120. One of the foremost members of the NCBE was Roy Torcaso, who had first come to national prominence because of the 1963 U.S. Supreme Court decision establishing the right not to be forced to swear to a god-bearing oath. Torcaso supported active euthanasia and believed that "babies born with obvious deformities or defects which will incapacitate the person (for instance blindness or missing limbs) should be allowed to die." Roy Torcaso to Frances Graves, 5 December 1977, NAC, MG31-K13, vol. 2, file 19.

121. "Humanist Concern for the Dying," n.d., NAC, MG31-K13, vol. 2, file 19.

122. "A Plea for Beneficent Euthanasia," *The Humanist* 34 (1974): 4–5.

123. Algernon Black, address to New York Society for Ethical Culture, 3 March 1963, cited in Larue, *Euthanasia and Religion*, 127–31. See also Algernon Black, "Euthanasia: To Live—Or Not to Live," n.d., PFC, Box C-2; "Algernon Black, Leader of Society for Ethical Culture, Is Dead," *New York Times*, 11 May 1993, B6. Another well-known Ethical Culture figure who defended euthanasia was Benjamin Miller. See Miller's "Euthanasia and the Ethics of Self-Fulfillment," address to the ESA, 19 January 1959, ESA *Bulletin*, March–April 1959, 2–4.

124. Humphry and Clement, *Freedom to Die*, 195, 271, 370.

125. Swallow, "Olive Ruth Russell," 99–100. In her later years she kept a poem, a parody of Psalm 23 that warned of the dangers of medical technology prolonging life, written by a Unitarian minister. See also Olive Ruth Russell, "Some Thoughts on Good Friday: Are We Immortal?" NAC, MG31-K13, vol. 1, file 10.

126. Author's telephone interview with Ruth Roettinger, 25 May 2001. See also Judy Flander, "She Knows Meaning of Euthanasia: Psychologist Relates a Personal Story," *Washington Star*, 29 December 1975; Olive Ruth Russell to Joseph Fletcher, 29 November 1977, NAC, MG31-K13, vol. 2, file 18; Olive Ruth Russell to Ann Landers, 30 December 1977, NAC, MG31-K13, vol. 2, file 16.

127. Brock Chisholm's (1896–1971) broad range of concerns encompassing euthanasia, population control, and sex education was indicative of the myriad currents intersecting with the right-to-die movement between World War II and the 1970s. Elected the World Health Organization's first director-general in 1948, and named Humanist of the Year in 1959 by the AHA, Chisholm echoed Russell's endorsement of voluntary and involuntary euthanasia. He too was an outspoken opponent of religious taboos about sex and reproduction, defending masturbation and contraception. In 1945 he created controversy in Canada when he accused parents who let their children believe in Santa Claus of permanently damaging their youngsters' emotional and cognitive development. Like Russell, Chisholm was a warm proponent of a United Nations–led world government and criticized the reluctance of industrial nations to curb population growth in the underdeveloped world through wide-scale sterilization programs, the main reason he became honorary president of the Human Better-

ment Association of America in the early 1960s. Horrified like so many by the Thalidomide disaster, in 1962 he proposed a committee of experts to adjudicate mercy killing of babies and adults. In his quest to achieve progress and human freedom, Chisholm, more so than Russell, believed that in solving social problems, individual liberty had to step aside in deference to science, medicine, technology, and state interests. He had no doubts that the job of determining what these interests were should be given to medical experts like himself. See Irving, *Brock Chisholm: Doctor to the World*. For Chisholm's defense of involuntary euthanasia, see ibid., 132. See also BC, MG30-B56, vol. 4, 1962 file; "Brock Chisholm Speaks Out," *Star Weekly Magazine*, 26 January 1963, 1–5. For Russell's acknowledgment of Chisholm's views on euthanasia, see Olive Ruth Russell, "Should Law Recognize a Right to Choose Death?" n.d., NAC, MG31-K13, vol. 2, file 16. Chisholm was one of the few to make the connection between thalidomide and euthanasia. Glick, *The Right to Die*, 73; Russell, *Freedom to Die*, 244.

128. Vogt and Whelpton were also members of Hugh Moore's AVS.

129. Minutes of the EEC board meeting, 16 January 1974, PFC, Box D-1.

130. A recent and revealing look at Moore's contributions to the population control and birth control movements is Critchlow's *Intended Consequences*, 4–5, 16–18, 20–33, 150–54.

131. For her reflections on trying to work with Moore, and his low opinion of the women in the family planning and euthanasia fields, see Frances Hand Ferguson's interview with James Reed, 3 June 1974, Schlesinger-Rockefeller Family Planning Oral History Project, Schlesinger Library, Radcliffe Institute, Harvard University, Cambridge, Mass., 46, 57. I wish to thank the Schlesinger Library for permission to quote from these materials. Ferguson was a member of both the ESA and HBAA/AVS.

132. Critchlow, *Intended Consequences*, 131.

133. As Moore stated in 1963, his interest in AVS "was not primarily domestic but rather international—in the hope that through sterilization something might be done to ease the social strains which bring on war." Hugh Moore to Ruth Proskauer Smith, 23 September 1963, HM, Series 3, Box 15, folder 6.

134. Hugh Moore, "Dear Friend Letter," November 1966, HM, Series 3, Box 15, folder 7. In 1968 he paid a New York City firm to develop advertisements that linked overpopulation to urban crime, poverty, and pollution. One ad, titled "Have You Been Mugged Today?" depicted what many believed was a young black man mugging a victim. The ads sparked charges of racism and accusations that Moore was blaming the poor for the "population explosion" and the crime it supposedly caused. Critchlow, *Intended Consequences*, 151.

135. In 1972 he gave $1,000 to Compulsory Birth Control for All Americans. See the comments of Edward J. Ennis, General Counsel of the ACLU, at the Association for Voluntary Sterilization's "National Conference on Voluntary Sterilization: Its Role in Averting World Starvation," 28 November 1967; Frank Rosa to Hugh Moore, 23 November 1967, HM, Series 3, Box 15, folder 3. Frederick

Jaffe of Planned Parenthood Federation of America and (later) the Alan Gutt-macher Institute wrote in 1970 that compulsory sterilization for all people with two children was necessary to slow U.S. population growth. *Family Planning Perspectives*, Special Supplement—U.S. Population Growth and Family Planning: A Review of the Literature, vol. 2, no. 4, October 1970, 24.

136. Moore was also a supporter of the abortion rights activist Lawrence Lader, who had worked for the Hugh Moore Fund in the 1960s. See Hugh Moore to Robert Willison, 1 September 1972, HM, Series 3, Box 2, folder 7.

137. Beginning with a $1,000 gift to the EEF in 1968, Moore provided matching funds up to $2,500 in 1969 and 1970. See "Contributions," HM, Series 3, Box 15, folder 29; Parker, Duryee, Zunino, Malone, and Carter to Mrs. Henry J. Mali, "Estate of Hugh Moore," 3 January 1974, PFC, Box E-1.

138. Shortly before he died, he informed the Atlanta Conference of the United Methodist Church that he supported his right to terminate his own life by whatever method he chose. Hugh Moore to the Atlanta Conference of the United Methodist Church, 2 May 1972, PFC, Box E-1.

139. See "Concern for Dying," JDR, Series 3, Subseries 3, Box 44, folder 262. For the negotiations among SRD, CFD, and Rockefeller, see John D. Rockefeller 3rd to Kay Mali, 21 May 1976, Florence Clothier to Joseph Fletcher, 6 March 1979, FC, Carton 1, folders 38, 157.

140. "Suicide Pact Preceded Deaths of Dr. Van Dusen and his Wife," *New York Times*, 26 February 1975, 1; "The Right to Die," *Saturday Review*, 14 June 1975, 4. Van Dusen's wife died on 28 January, but Van Dusen vomited the pills they had taken jointly and lingered for fifteen more days before dying on 13 February of a heart ailment.

141. Russell, *Freedom to Die*, 396 (1977 ed.).

142. Russell, *Freedom to Die*, 8 (preface to the 1977 ed.) See also Russell, "Freedom to Choose Death."

Chapter 5

1. Glick, *The Right to Die*, 83–87.

2. Kay Mali, transcript of EEC board meeting, 17 April 1974, PFC, Box D-1.

3. Donald W. McKinney to Mrs. Henry W. (A-J) Rock Levinson, 15 December 1976, PFC, Box D-1.

4. Donald W. McKinney to "Fellow Unitarian-Universalists," 3 November 1970, PFC, Box D-1.

5. Donald W. McKinney, *Whose Life Is It Anyway?* (Brooklyn: First Unitarian Church, n.d.) 2.

6. Telephone interview with Donald McKinney, 21 December 1999.

7. McKinney to Mrs. Henry W. (A-J) Rock Levinson, 15 December 1976, PFC, Box D-1.

8. The SRD bylaws articulated the "need for euthanasia whether by terminations of medical procedures or positive action under adequate safeguard." Elizabeth Halsey to Joseph Fletcher, 2 January 1975, PFC, Box D-1.

9. Minutes of the EEC board meeting, 17 January 1973, PFC, Box D-1.

10. Joseph Fletcher, *To Live and to Die: When, Why, and How* (New York: Springer-Verlag, 1973), 113. Reprinted as "Ethics and Euthanasia," in Horan and Mall, eds., *Death, Dying, and Euthanasia*, 293–304, quote on 293.

11. "Transcript," EEC board meeting, 17 April 1974, p. 7, PFC, Box D-1.

12. Minutes of the EEC board meeting, 15 May 1974, PFC, Box D-1.

13. Matters simply had reached the point, Mali declared, where the operations of both organizations were "impair[ed]." "President's Report," 6 December 1975, PFC, Box D-1. The issue became moot when the EEC changed its own name in 1978 to CFD, due to the wide perception that euthanasia was the same as mercy killing. A-J Rock Levinson, "Memorandum" to EEC board members, 3 March 1977, PFC, Box D-1.

14. Minutes of the EEC "brainstorming session," 24 March 1977, PFC, Box D-1.

15. Minutes of the SRD annual meeting, 15 December 1978, PFC, Box D-1. Mali also informed the SRD of CFD's board decision that officers of either organization serving on both boards be requested to resign from the board of the organization of which they are not officers. Sidney Rosoff, "To the Members of the Board of Directors of the Society for the Right to Die," 30 March 1979, PFC, Box D-1.

16. Minutes of CFD board meeting, 13 June 1979, 12 September 1979, PFC, Box D-1.

17. Mrs. Henry J. (Kay) Mali to Florence Clothier, 17 January 1979, FC, Carton 2, folder 113; Kay Mali, untitled CFD memorandum, 19 September 1979, PFC, Box D-1.

18. Florence Clothier, "Confronting Mortality: When Is the 'Quality of Mercy' Strained?" *Perspectives on Aging* 4 (1975): 3–7. Her emphasis.

19. Florence Clothier to Claiborne Pell, 24 August 1976, FC, Carton 1, folder 35.

20. Clothier, "Confronting Mortality."

21. Florence Clothier, letter to *Life*, 17 January 1972, FC, Carton 1, folder 40.

22. Florence Clothier to Kay Mali, 5 February 1973, FC, Carton 1, folder 38.

23. Florence Clothier to Mali, 25 February 1977, FC, Carton 1, folder 34.

24. Clothier may have expressed unconventional opinions about involuntary euthanasia, but movement members remained fond of her. In fact, Clothier continued to serve on CFD's advisory committee after the split between the two groups in 1980.

25. Rosoff made his support for active euthanasia clear at the Third International Conference on Voluntary Euthanasia and Suicide, held at Oxford, England, 11–14 September 1980. Frank Dungey, "EXIT Newsletter No. 6," April 1981, 11, PFC, Box F-3. Rosoff recounted his history in the euthanasia movement in his 17 May 1990 letter to Bernard Toomin, assistant attorney general of New York State, PFC,

uncatalogued. To Derek Humphry, Rosoff "philosophically agreed" with Hemlock's advocacy of physician-assisted suicide even while he was a member of the SRD. Author's telephone interview with Derek Humphry, 13 December 2001.

26. Telephone interview with Mary Meyer, 14 September 2000. Smith's parents were Joseph M. Proskauer, a noted jurist and Democratic Party insider, and Alice (Naumburg) Proskauer, a New York City community activist.

27. McGreevy, "Thinking on One's Own," 97–131.

28. Guttmacher served on the ESA advisory council until the late 1960s. According to Smith, Guttmacher occasionally euthanized "monstrosities" on his maternity ward. Interview with Ruth Proskauer Smith, 11 November 2000, New York, N.Y.; Ruth Proskauer Smith, "Remarks by Ruth P. Smith at SRD's 50th Anniversary Celebration," 7 December 1988, PFC, uncatalogued.

29. She served as HBAA executive director until 1964. Interview with Ruth Proskauer Smith, 11 November 2000, New York, N.Y. See also SWHA, SW 15.1, Box 15, Fletcher Folder, Box 16, Guttmacher Folder, Box 18, Ruth Proskauer Smith Folder.

30. "Remarks by Ruth P. Smith," 9; interview with Ruth Proskauer Smith, November 2000.

31. "Remarks by Ruth P. Smith," 7–8, 9.

32. Quarrels led to Smith's departure from the HBAA in 1964 and the Association for the Study of Abortion in 1966. See the comments of Kurt Borchardt, Kay Mali, and Ruth P. Smith, "Verbatim Notes," board meeting of the SRD, 13 March 1979, PFC, Box D-1; Florence Clothier to Alice Mehling, 27 March 1979; Florence Clothier to Ruth Smith, 27 March 1979, PFC, Box D-1; telephone interview with Mary Meyer, 14 September 2000, in which Smith was described as "very pro-assisted suicide" and a "very difficult woman." For comments on Rosoff and his contributions to "personal disputes," see Supreme Court of the State of New York, County of New York, "Memorandum of Law in Support of Petitioners' Application for an Order Approving Plan of Merger and in Opposition to Proposed Intervenors' Motion," 17 September 1990, 7. What seems to have accelerated the break between CFD and the SRD was a policy proposal written by Clothier and read by Ruth Smith at the SRD board's 15 December 1978 meeting. It encouraged discussion of euthanasia for those "doomed to a crib existence" as a long-term policy option the SRD ought to consider. Minutes of the SRD board meeting, 15 December 1978, PFC, Box D-1. According to Derek Humphry, Smith, like Rosoff, belonged to the Hemlock Society at the same time she was a member of the SRD. Author's telephone interview with Derek Humphry, 13 December 2001.

33. Further affiliation with the SRD meant not only difficulties in fund-raising for CFD; it also meant that CFD would encounter resistance in its efforts to organize seminars and participate in conferences with liberal Catholics, as occurred at the Second International Euthanasia Conference in San Francisco in 1978. See the comments of A-J Rock Levinson and Donald McKinney, n.d., FC, Carton 1, folder 113.

34. William J. Woodcock, "Request by SRD for CFD Grant," Memorandum to CFD's board of directors, 13 October 1978, PFC, Box D-1.

35. Moore's former wife, the SRD's Louise Van Vleck, asserted that Moore had wanted his money to be used for "activist work," not for CFD "studies." "There has to be someone to stick his neck out," Moore is reputed to have said. Comments of Louise Van Vleck, "Verbatim Notes," board meeting of the SRD, 13 March 1979, 4, PFC, Box D-1. Tempers also flared when CFD tried to tempt "Dear Abby" to take its side. However, by 1980, Abby and Sidney Rosoff had become friends by working together over the years. "Dear Abby," whose views were perhaps closer to CFD's position than the SRD's, remained loyal to the SRD. After the split, "Dear Abby" listed only the SRD's address in her columns when readers requested information about death with dignity. According to Marjorie Zucker, Abby "saved" the SRD in the 1980s. Telephone interview with Marjorie Zucker, 2 November 2000.

36. Richard Wasserman to Mrs. Henry J. Mali, 9 October 1979, PFC, Box D-1.

37. Humphry and Wickett, *The Right to Die*, 112; telephone interview with Donald McKinney, 21 December 1999.

38. Comments of Joseph Fletcher, "Verbatim Notes," board meeting of the SRD, 13 March 1979, 4; minutes of the SRD board meeting 15 December 1978, PFC, Box D-1.

39. CFD had decided that it had reached "the end of its first period of growth and development," and a growing number of SRD members felt the same. A-J Rock Levinson, "Annual Report to [CFD's] Board of Directors," September 1978, PFC, Box D-1.

40. Comments of Kay Mali, "Verbatim Notes," board meeting of the SRD, 13 March 1979, PFC, Box D-1, 1.

41. Filene, *In the Arms of Others*, 22–25.

42. Ramsey, *Ethics at the Edges of Life*, 294. Kamisar's speech was essentially the same he delivered in 1977 at State University of New York at Buffalo, titled "A Life Not (Or No Longer) Worth Living: Are We Deciding the Issue Without Facing It?" For an account of the speech, see *Quadrangle Notes* (University of Michigan Law School) 22 (1978): 3–4.

43. Filene, *In the Arms of Others*, 73.

44. Kurt Borchardt to Alice Mehling, 20 April 1976, FC, Carton 1, folder 34.

45. Filene, *In the Arms of Others*, 106–7; Keith Cassidy, "The Right to Life Movement," in Critchlow, ed., *The Politics of Abortion and Birth Control in Historical Perspective*, 128–59.

46. Critchlow, *Intended Consequences*, 200.

47. For how euthanasia was "becoming more intertwined with abortion," and the "worried" reaction of the SRD, see " 'Right to Die': Second Battle for Abortion Foes," *New York Times*, 31 July 1990, A1; Julie A. Grimstad and Mary Senander, "Have Our Religious Leaders Abandoned the Least Brethren?" *The Church World*, 14 January 1988, 5. See also Allitt, *Catholic Intellectuals and Conservative Politics in America, 1950–1985*, 193. Activists such as Ruth Smith, Joseph Fletcher, and Flor-

ence Clothier believed that if the state had no right to tell a woman how to control her fertility, it had no right to stop someone from controlling his or her death. This continues to be the position of the pro-abortion National Organization for Women (NOW) and Planned Parenthood Federation of America, which insist that "choice is choice." Smith, *Forced Exit*, 210. In the words of Hemlock Society cofounder Derek Humphry, "[m]ost people who believe in abortion also believe in voluntary euthanasia, as a generalization." Derek Humphry, "Supreme Court Accepts Cruzan Case: To Rule on Right to Die," *Medical Ethics Advisor* 5 (1989): 97–101, quote on 99.

48. For an account of the battle over the 1976 California Natural Death Act, see Filene, *In the Arms of Others*, 98–105; Glick, *The Right to Die*, 93–98.

49. Handwritten note of Senator Edward Kennedy to Florence Clothier, n.d. (likely 1981), FC, Addenda, Box 1, folder 9. See also Evelyn Ames Davis to Sidney Wanzer, 17 July 1980, PFC, uncatalogued, for comments about "the viciousness of the Right to Lifers at this particular time."

50. Olive Ruth Russell to Frances Graves, 21 September 1978, NAC, MG31-K13, vol. 2, file 18. One SRD member lamented in 1979 that the feuding between CFD and the SRD played "into the hands of the Right-to-Life organization." Comments of Bess Dana, "Verbatim Notes," SRD board meeting, 13 March 1979, p. 2, PFC, Box D-1.

51. Frances Graves to Olive Ruth Russell, 6 February 1976, NAC, MG31-K13, vol. 2, file 19; Frances Graves to Roy Torcaso, 24 August 1978, NAC, MG31-K13, vol. 2, file 18.

52. Rosoff's presence as its president was an important stumbling block. In the midst of the split between the two groups, CFD officials were reluctant to belong to an organization headed by one of the chief instigators of the lawsuit.

53. "Booklet on Self-Deliverance: Press Statement by Larry Hill, the Acting Chairman," 11 August 1980, PFC, Box F-3; "British 'Right to Die' Group Plans to Publish a Manual on Suicide," *New York Times*, 7 March 1980, A18; "British Guide to Suicide Is Blocked by Legal Perils," *New York Times*, 12 August 1980, A11; "EXIT's Guide to Suicide Starts a Storm," *London Observer*, 14 September 1980. The Scottish chapter of EXIT, however, went ahead and published a suicide guide, calling their London counterparts "moral cowards." "Publish and Be Damned?" *Economist*, 30 August 1980, 45.

54. Donald McKinney to Adrienne van Till, 6 November 1981, PFC, Box F-4; "Statement from the President of Concern for Dying Re: The Third International Euthanasia Conference," September 1980, PFC, Box F-3. See also "EXIT Verdict Is Blow to Euthanasia Campaign," *Times* (London), 31 October 1981, 3; Otlowski, *Voluntary Euthanasia and the Common Law*, 270–71; Humphry and Wickett, *The Right to Die*, 127–36.

55. See CFD's report on the 1984 Nice International Conference, at which "[i]t was apparent that the European view differs greatly from ours with regard to active euthanasia, suicide, and who should make treatment decisions in terminal ill-

ness. Regarding the latter, Europeans tend to leave decision making to the doc-tors." Minutes of the CFD board meeting, 3 October 1984, PFC, uncatalogued. See also A-J Rock Levinson to Derek Humphry, 5 February 1985, PFC, Box F-4, in which Levinson asserts that some in the World Federation "advocate what, in this country and in many others, is clearly 'murder.' " For impressions of the Nice Conference from an anti-euthanasia activist, see Marker, *Deadly Compassion*, 49–64.

56. In his most recent account of the founding of Hemlock, Humphry appears to give equal credit to University of Southern California professor of religious stud-ies Gerald Larue for starting the group. See Humphry and Clement, *Freedom to Die*, 114–15.

57. Anne Fadiman, "Death News: Requiem for the Hemlock Quarterly," *Harpers* 288 (April 1994): 75.

58. In 1988 Sidney Rosoff declared that the origins of the ESA "are what Hemlock represents today." Marker, *Deadly Compassion*, 96.

59. Marker, *Deadly Compassion*, 230; Woodman, *Last Rights*, 122–26. Wickett's emphasis.

60. Author's telephone interview with Derek Humphry, 13 December 2001.

61. Diane M. Gianelli, "Oregon Voters Face 'RX-Only' Suicide Initiative," *American Medical News*, 12 September 1994, 1, 34. Cited in Annas, *Some Choice*, 220.

62. Humphry and Clement, *Freedom to Die*, 339, 340, 342, 347, 348. For a criticism that focuses on this aspect of Humphry's approach to euthanasia, see Sherwin B. Nuland, "The Right to Live," *The New Republic*, 2 November 1998, 29–35, quote on 33.

63. New York State Task Force on Life and the Law, *When Death Is Sought*, 30–32. See also Herbert Hendin, *Suicide in America*, rev. ed. (New York: Norton, 1995), 81–82, 132. Cited in Filene, *In the Arms of Others*, 187.

64. Nuland, *How We Die*, 1172–79; Mirko Grmek, *History of AIDS: Emergence and Origin of a Modern Pandemic* (Princeton: Princeton University Press, 1990), 32, 41; In-stitute of Medicine, National Academy of Sciences, *Confronting AIDS: Update 1988* (Washington, D.C.: National Academy Press, 1988), 51; Filene, *In the Arms of Others*, 150.

65. *When Death Is Sought*, 28–30; Annas, *Some Choice*, 231. See also Thomas A. Preston and Ralph Mero, "Observations Concerning Terminally Ill Patients Who Choose Suicide," *Journal of Pharmaceutical Care and Pain Symptom Control* 4 (1996): 183–92.

66. Woodman, *Last Rights*, 191–92. See also Lee R. Slome et al., "Physician-Assisted Suicide and Patients with Human Immunodeficiency Virus Disease," *New England Journal of Medicine* 336 (1997): 417–21; "Changing the Rules on Dying," *U.S. News and World Report*, 9 July 1990, 22.

67. *Evans v. Bellevue Hospital*, No. 16536/87, New York Supreme Court, N.Y. County, 27 July 1987.

68. "Has He a Right to Die?" *New York Daily News*, 15 July 1987.

69. "Presidential Panel Holds Hearings on 'Right to Die,' " *New York Times*, 12 April

1981, 24; Telephone interview with Donald McKinney, 21 December 1999; Mc-Kinney personal communication, 1 August 2001. Derek Humphry and Ann Wickett alleged that the SRD believed McKinney and CFD had "sabotaged" any attempts at legislation. Humphry and Wickett, *The Right to Die*, 114n. McKinney claims that because they were so persuaded by his testimony, Alex Capron, the President Commission's director, and Joanne Lynn, the commission's medical director, joined the CFD board. See President's Commission for the Study of Ethical Problems in Medicine and Biomedical and Behavioral Research, *Summing Up: Final Report on Studies of the Ethical and Legal Problems in Medicine and Biomedical and Behavioral Research* (Washington, D.C.: U.S. Government Printing Office, 1983).

70. Materials regarding the Dax Cowart story can be found in PFC, Box B-15.
71. "Love and Let Die," *Time*, 19 March 1990, 65.
72. William Steel, "Lives in the Balance," PFC, Box B-15.
73. Donald McKinney, CFD meeting of the advisory committee on the Dax Cowart film, 12–14 November 1982, PFC, Box B-15.
74. Concern for Dying, "Suicide: A Need for New Thinking," PFC, Box F-3.
75. Derek Humphry to Donald McKinney, 28 January 1985, PFC, Box F-4. See also A-J Rock Levinson to Derek Humphry, 5 February 1985; Donald McKinney to Derek Humphry, 7 February 1985, PFC, Box F-4.
76. Minutes of CFD board meeting, 20 April 1981, PFC, uncatalogued.
77. Then there was Estelle Browning, who, despite having drawn up a living will in 1985 at the age of eighty-five, was paralyzed and attached to a feeding tube two and a half years later because her Florida physicians and the nurses at her nursing home, reasoning her death was not "imminent," decided to obey a state requirement that nursing homes feed all patients. Joseph Carey, "The Faulty Promise of 'Living Wills'," *U.S. News and World Report*, 24 July 1989, 63–64.
78. Filene, *In the Arms of Others*, 157, 179.
79. Quote is from Tom Horkan, executive director of the Florida Catholic Conference. See "Presidential Panel Holds Hearings on 'Right to Die,'" *New York Times*, 12 April 1981; Garrett, "The Last Civil Right?" 185. For the living will's limitations, see Robert Barry, "What a Living Will Does Not Protect You Against," *New York Times*, 21 December 1985, 26; Filene, *In the Arms of Others*, 159–60, 184–85. Not all Catholic theologians opposed the living will, a fact that Sidney Rosoff and the SRD exploited in their own literature. Sidney Rosoff, "Dear Friend," undated, PFC, uncatalogued. See John J. Paris and Richard A. McCormick, "Living Will Legislation: Reconsidered," *America*, 5 September 1981, 86–89.
80. Joseph Fletcher to Fenella Rouse, 20 April 1989, PFC, uncatalogued.
81. Mary Ellen Avery to Fenella Rouse, 19 April 1989, PFC, uncatalogued.
82. W. F. Rogers III to Evan R. Collins, Jr., 12 February 1988, PFC, uncatalogued.
83. Minutes of the SRD board meeting, 9 August 1989; minutes of the SRD board meeting, 17 February 1988, PFC, uncatalogued.
84. Ruth Proskauer Smith, "Backgrounder for the Feb. 21 1987 'Retreat,'" PFC, uncatalogued, 5.

85. Filene, *In the Arms of Others*, 108–14, 119–24.

86. "Report of the Subcommittee on the Severely Impaired Newborn," c. 1983, PFC, uncatalogued; minutes of the 6 June 1984 SRD executive committee meeting, PFC, uncatalogued. For a sharp criticism of endowing an infant with a right to die, see Nat Hentoff, "The Awful Privacy of Baby Doe," *The Atlantic Monthly*, January 1985, 54–62.

87. Lamm and his defenders claimed he had been quoted out of context, and that he merely was trying to draw attention to the allocation of limited resources to those who were terminally ill and had little quality of life. See Richard D. Lamm, "Long Time Dying," *New Republic*, 27 August 1984, 20–25; "Question: Who Will Play God?" *Time*, 9 April 1984, 68; Evan R. Collins, Jr., "To Die or Not to Die," *New York Times*, 4 April 1984; Richard D. Lamm, "Saving a Few, Sacrificing Many—At Great Cost," *New York Times*, 2 August 1989. However, Lamm did endorse Humphry's *Final Exit*.

88. Sanford Schwartz, "Active Euthanasia and Assisted Suicide," April 1985, PFC, uncatalogued. The heavy dependency of the SRD on "Dear Abby" was discussed at the 12 April 1989 board meeting, PFC, uncatalogued.

89. Minutes of the SRD board meeting, 13 March 1985, PFC, uncatalogued; Sanford Schwartz, memo, January 1987, PFC, uncatalogued.

90. "Address by Dr. Joseph Fletcher, SRD Annual Dinner Meeting, Harvard Club, December 9, 1986," PFC, Box F-4. His emphasis.

91. Joseph Fletcher, quoted by Ruth P. Smith, "Backgrounder for February 21, 1987 'Retreat,' " PFC, uncatalogued, 5.

92. Smith, "Backgrounder," 5.

93. Sidney H. Wanzer, S. James Adelstein, Ronald E. Cranford, et al., "The Physician's Responsibility Toward Hopelessly Ill Patients," *The New England Journal of Medicine* 310 (1984): 955–59.

94. Sidney H. Wanzer, Daniel D. Federman, S. James Adelstein, et al., "The Physician's Responsibility Toward Hopelessly Ill Patients: A Second Look," *The New England Journal of Medicine* 320 (1989): 844–49. See also "Correspondence," *The New England Journal of Medicine* 321 (1989): 975–78; David Orentlicher, "Physician Participation in Assisted Suicide," *Journal of the American Medical Association* 262 (1989): 1844–45.

95. "Jeff Buckner, M.D., Statement," undated (c. 1989); Memo of Sanford Schwartz, 11 May 1989, p. 1, PFC, uncatalogued.

96. Carol Farkas to Alice Mehling, undated (c. 1987); "Memo to SRD Board from Sia Arnason," 23 January 1986; minutes of SRD board meeting, 14 June 1989; minutes of SRD board meeting, 10 May 1989, PFC, uncatalogued.

97. Minutes of the 15 January 1986 SRD board meeting, PFC, uncatalogued.

98. Ruth Roettinger to Bernard Toomin, 12 May 1990, PFC, uncatalogued.

99. Minutes of the 9 August 1989 and 15 November 1989 SRD board meetings, PFC, uncatalogued.

100. Minutes of the 31 January 1990 SRD board meeting, PFC, uncatalogued.

101. "Memorandum of Law . . . ," 3.

102. Minutes of the SRD board meeting, 11 December 1989, PFC, uncatalogued.

103. "Minutes of the Special Meeting of the Voting Members of the SRD," 16 April 1990, PFC, uncatalogued.

104. Sidney Rosoff to Bernard Toomin, 17 May 1990, PFC, uncatalogued; Supreme Court of the State of New York, County of New York, "Settlement Agreement," June 1991, PFC, uncatalogued; author's interview with Ruth Proskauer Smith, 11 November 2000, New York, N.Y.

105. Partnership for Caring, Inc., "Position Statement: 'Leaving Our Differences at the Door,' " http://www.partnershipforcaring.org.

106. Author's telephone interview with Derek Humphry, 13 December 2001.

Chapter 6

1. The only exception to Oregon in U.S. history was Texas, where until 1973 there was no law prohibiting the aiding and abetting of suicide. See H. Tristam Engelhardt, Jr., Edmund L. Erde, and John Moskop, "Euthanasia in Texas: A Little Known Experiment," *Hospital Physician*, September 1976: 30–31.

2. Author's telephone interview with Derek Humphry, 13 December 2001.

3. "To Feed or Not to Feed?" *Time*, 31 March 1986, 60; "Changing the Rules on Dying," *U.S. News and World Report*, 9 July 1990, 22–23.

4. Filene, *In the Arms of Others*, 168–83.

5. Zucker, ed., *The Right to Die Debate*, 190–201, quote on 192.

6. Ellen Goodman, "The High-Tech Twilight Zone," *Boston Globe*, 28 June 1990; "State Supreme Court's Cruzan Ruling Certain to Affect Nation," *Springfield News-Leader*, 20 November 1988; Linda Greenhouse, "Liberty to Reject Life," *New York Times*, 27 June 1990, A16.

7. Humphry and Clement, *Freedom to Die*, 124. See also Larson and Amundsen, *A Different Death*, 184.

8. "It's Over, Debbie," *JAMA* 259 (1988): 272.

9. Charles Krauthammer, "The 'Death' of 'Debbie,' " *Washington Post*, 26 February 1988. A similar view was expressed in Willard Gaylin, Leon R. Kass, Edmund R. Pellegrino, and Mark Siegler, "Doctors Must Not Kill," in Moreno, ed., *Arguing Euthanasia*, 33–36, quote on 34. See also Garrett, "The Last Civil Right?" 205; Isabel Wilkerson, "Essay on Mercy Killing Reflects Conflict on Ethics for Physicians and Journalists," *New York Times*, 23 February 1988, A16; Isabel Wilkerson, "Judge Stalls Inquiry into a Mercy-Killing Case," *New York Times*, 19 March 1988, A15.

10. "Letters," *JAMA* 259 (1988): 2094–98; Kenneth L. Vaux, "Debbie's Dying: Mercy Killing and the Good Death," *JAMA* 259 (1988): 2140–41; George D. Lundberg, " 'It's Over, Debbie' and the Euthanasia Debate," *JAMA* 259 (1988): 2142–43.

11. Michael Betzold, "The Selling of Doctor Death," *New Republic*, 26 May 1997, 22–28.

12. "The Doctor's Suicide Van," *Newsweek*, 18 June 1990, 46–49.

13. In fact, of the sixty-nine patients Kevorkian helped to die up to 1998, only seventeen were actually dying before they sought his assistance. Lisa Priest, "Most Kevorkian Suicides Weren't Terminally Ill," *The Globe and Mail*, 7 December 2000.

14. Hemlock Society, Press Release, 26 October 1989. Cited in Garrett, "The Last Civil Right?" 213. See also Jack Lessenberry, "Death and the Matron," *Esquire* 127 (April 1997): 80–85, 130–31.

15. Humphry and Clement, *Freedom to Die*, 136.

16. Stephanie Gutmann, "Death and the Maiden," *New Republic*, 24 June 1996, 20–28.

17. Woodman, *Last Rights*, 146–48.

18. "Voters Turn Down Mercy Killing Idea," *New York Times*, 7 November 1991, B16.

19. Garrett, "The Last Civil Right?" 192–94.

20. Woodman, *Last Rights*, 143–44. The split between Mero and Hemlock was "amicable." Half the members of the Compassion board in 1993 also sat on the local Hemlock board, and the two organizations had adjacent office space. Lisa Belkin, "There's No Simple Suicide," *New York Times*, 14 November 1993, 50–56, 74–75, quote on 54.

21. Lawrence K. Altman, "A How-To Book on Suicide Surges to Top of Best-Seller List in Week," *New York Times*, 9 August 1991.

22. Garrett, "The Last Civil Right?" 248; Annas, *Some Choice*, 214–15. See also New York State Task Force on Life and the Law, *When Death Is Sought*, 133–34. For Dutch euthanasia, see P. J. Van der Maas et al., "Euthanasia and Other Medical Decisions Concerning the End of Life," *Lancet* 338 (1991): 669–74; P. J. Van der Maas et al., "Euthanasia, Physician-Assisted Suicide, and Other Medical Practices Involving the End of Life in the Netherlands, 1990–1995," *New England Journal of Medicine* 335 (1996): 1699–1705; G. Van der Wal et al., "Evaluation of the Notification Procedure for Physician-Assisted Suicide in the Netherlands," *New England Journal of Medicine* 335 (1996): 1706–11. For American reactions to these studies, see Herbert Hendin, Chris Rutenfrans, and Zbigniew Zylicz, "Physician-Assisted Suicide and Euthanasia in the Netherlands," *JAMA* 277 (1997): 1720–22; Marcia Angell, "Euthanasia in the Netherlands—Good News or Bad?" *New England Journal of Medicine* 335 (1996): 1676–98. Defenders of Dutch euthanasia contend that in the majority of nonvoluntary euthanasia cases assistance in dying was at least *discussed* with the patients, that the decision was rarely the physician's solely, and that in almost all the cases the patients were in the last stages of dying. Woodman, *Last Rights*, 83–84.

23. Garrett, "The Last Civil Right?" 251–52. A Louis Harris and Associates 1987 poll, commissioned by the Harvard Community Health Plan, showed that 66 percent of doctors considered it wrong for a physician to comply with patients' wishes to end their lives, in contrast to 38 percent of the general public. Wilkerson, "Essay on Mercy Killing," A16.

24. "Foes of Euthanasia Measure Gain Ground in Washington State," *New York Times*, 4 November 1991, A16; Garrett, "The Last Civil Right?" 271.

25. Timothy Quill, "Death and Dignity: A Case of Individualized Decision-Making," *New England Journal of Medicine* 324 (1991): 691–94. See also Lawrence K. Altman, "Doctor Says He Gave Patient Drug to Help Her Commit Suicide," *New York Times*, 7 March 1991, A1; Lawrence K. Altman, "Jury Declines to Indict a Doctor Who Said He Aided in a Suicide," *New York Times*, 27 July 1991, A1.

26. Quill, *Caring for Patients at the End of Life: Facing An Uncertain Future Together* (New York: Oxford University Press, 2001), 132–47, 161–62, 182–84; author's telephone interview with Timothy Quill, 13 November 2001. See also Zucker, *The Right to Die Debate*, 282–95.

27. Nuland, *How We Die*, 154–56.

28. Humphry and Clement, *Freedom to Die*, 240.

29. Transcript of "Yes on 16" advertisement aired on various stations, beginning October 24, 1994. Quoted in Smith, *Forced Exit*, 118–19.

30. Author's telephone interview with Derek Humphry, 13 December 2001; Humphry and Clement, *Freedom to Die*, 253.

31. Humphry and Clement, *Freedom to Die*, 248. See also Derek Humphry, "Oregon's Assisted Suicide Law Gives No Sure Comfort to Dying," *New York Times*, 3 December 1994, 22.

32. "Reno Sides With Assisted-Suicide Law," *Globe and Mail* (Toronto), 6 June 1998, A19; "U.S. House Moves to Kill Oregon's Doctor-Assisted Suicide Law, *National Post*, 28 October 1999, A12; "Ashcroft's Crackdown Outrages Many in Oregon," *USA Today*, 12 November 2001, 4A; "As Suicide Approvals Rise in Oregon, Half Goes Unused," *New York Times*, 7 February 2002.

33. Annas, *Some Choice*, 224.

34. Linda Greenhouse, "Before the Court, the Sanctity of Life and Death," *New York Times*, 5 January 1997, 4–5.

35. "Suicides or Executions: Physicians Should Not Participate," *American Medical News*, 4 December 2000 (amednews.com).

36. Wilfred M. McClay, *The Masterless: Self and Society in Modern America* (Chapel Hill: University of North Carolina Press, 1994), 291, 295.

37. The New York State Task Force on Life and the Law, *When Death Is Sought: Assisted Suicide and Euthanasia in the Medical Context* (New York: New York State Task Force on Life and the Law, 1994), xiii, 118. Justice Kennedy is quoted in Annas, *Some Choice*, 240. The Task Force was important because it was "the only long-standing, government-sponsored multi-disciplinary group that has carefully studied the issue of physician assisted suicide with a view toward proposing legislation." Ibid., 240.

38. T. Egan, "In Oregon, Opening a New Front in the World of Medicine," *New York Times*, 6 November 1997, A26; David J. Garrow, "The Oregon Trail," *New York Times*, 6 November 1997, A27.

39. Author's telephone interview with Derek Humphry, 13 December 2001.

40. John Ostheimer, "The Polls: Changing Attitudes Toward Euthanasia," *Public Opinion Quarterly* 44 (1980): 123–28; "73% Polled Back Right to Die," *USA Today*,

3 January 1984, 3A; Glick, *The Right to Die*, 79–85; Gina Kolata, "Withholding Care from Patients: Boston Case Asks, Who Decides?" *New York Times*, 3 April 1995, A1. In a survey in the *New England Journal of Medicine*, published in 1996, 60 percent of Oregon doctors admitted they should be able to help terminal patients die. Michael D. Lemonick, "Defining the Right to Die," *Time*, 15 April 1996, 58.

41. Humphry and Clement, *Freedom to Die*, 190; author's telephone interview with Timothy Quill, 13 November 2001.

42. Glick, *The Right to Die*, 85.

43. Ezekiel Emanuel, "Whose Right to Die?" *Atlantic Monthly*, March 1997, 73–79, 74.

44. Yale Kamisar, "The Rise and Fall of the 'Right' to Assisted Suicide," in Foley and Hendin, eds., *The Case Against Assisted Suicide*, 92.

45. New York State Task Force on Life and the Law, *When Death Is Sought*, 102–3.

46. Filene, *In the Arms of Others*, 159–60.

Bibliography

Primary Sources

Harry Elmer Barnes Collection, American Heritage Center, University of Wyoming, Laramie

Florence Clothier Papers, Schlesinger Library, Radcliffe Institute, Harvard University

Robert Latou Dickinson Papers, Francis Countway Library, Harvard University

Engenderhealth Papers, Social Welfare History Archives, University of Minnesota, Minneapolis

Eugenics Society Archives, Contemporary Medical Archives Center, Wellcome Institute for the History of Medicine, London

Schlesinger-Rockefeller Family Planning Oral History Project, Schlesinger Library, Radcliffe Institute, Harvard University

Horace M. Kallen Papers, American Jewish Archives, Cincinnati, Ohio

Hugh Moore Fund Collection, Seeley G. Mudd Library, Princeton University

Partnership for Caring, Inc., Records (formerly the Euthanasia Society of America), Lewis Advertising, Baltimore

Inez Celia Philbrick File, State Archives and Manuscript Division, Nebraska State Historical Society, Lincoln

John D. Rockefeller 3rd Papers, Rockefeller Archive Center, Tarrytown, N.Y.

Olive Ruth Russell Collection, National Archives of Canada, Ottawa

Ruth Proskauer Smith Papers, Schlesinger Library, Radcliffe Institute, Harvard University

Voluntary Euthanasia Society Archives, Contemporary Medical Archives Center, Wellcome Institute for the History of Medicine, London

Interviews

Annas, George, telephone, 28 June 2001

Humphry, Derek, telephone, 13 December 2001

Kaplan, Karen, telephone, 8 December 1999

McKinney, Donald, telephone, 21 December 1999

Meyer, Mary, telephone, 4 September 2000

Quill, Timothy, telephone, 13 November 2001

Roettinger, Ruth, telephone, 25 May 2001

Smith, Ruth Proskauer, 11 November 2000

Zucker, Marjorie, telephone, 2 November 2000

Books and Articles

Adler, Felix. *An Ethical Philosophy of Life: Presented in Its Main Outlines.* 1919. Repr., Hicksville, N.Y.: The Regina Press, 1975.

Alexander, Leo. "Medical Science under Dictatorship." *New England Journal of Medicine* 241 (1949): 39–47.

Allitt, Patrick. *Catholic Intellectuals and Conservative Politics in America, 1950–1985.* Ithaca, N.Y.: Cornell University Press, 1993.

Aly, Götz, Peter Chroust, and Christian Pross. *Cleansing the Fatherland: Nazi Medicine and Racial Hygiene.* Trans. Belinda Cooper. Baltimore: Johns Hopkins University Press, 1994.

Annas, George J. "The Supreme Court, Privacy, and Abortion," *New England Journal of Medicine* 321 (1989): 1200–1203.

———. *Some Choice: Law, Medicine, and the Market.* New York: Oxford University Press, 1998.

Appleman, Philip, ed. *Darwin: A Norton Critical Edition.* New York: Norton, 1979.

Bailyn, Bernard, Robert Dallek, David Brion Davis, David Herbert Donald, John C. Thomas, and Gordon S. Wood, eds. *The Great Republic: A History of the American People.* 3rd ed. Lexington, Mass.: D.C. Health and Co., 1985.

Barnes, Harry Elmer. *The Twilight of Christianity.* New York: Vanguard Press, 1929.

Benedict, Susan, and Jochen Kuhla. "Nurses' Participation in the Euthanasia Programs of Nazi Germany," *Western Journal of Nursing Research* 21 (1999): 246–64.

Blanshard, Paul. *American Freedom and Catholic Power.* Boston: Beacon Press, 1950.

Bowler, Peter J. *The Non-Darwinian Revolution: Reinterpreting a Historical Myth.* Baltimore: Johns Hopkins University Press, 1992.

Broberg, Gunnar, and Nils Roll-Hansen, eds. *Eugenics and the Welfare State: Sterilization Policy in Denmark, Sweden, Norway, and Finland.* East Lansing: Michigan State University Press, 1996.

Burleigh, Michael. *Death and Deliverance: "Euthanasia" in Germany, 1900–1945.* Cambridge: Cambridge University Press, 1994.

Burnham, John C. "American Medicine's Golden Age: What Happened to it?" *Science* 215 (1982): 1474–79.

———. *Paths into American Culture: Psychology, Medicine, and Morals.* Philadelphia: Temple University Press, 1988.

Chesler, Ellen. *Woman of Valour: Margaret Sanger and the Birth Control Movement in America.* New York: Simon and Schuster, 1992.

Claeys, Gregory. "The 'Survival of the Fittest' and the Origins of Social Darwinism," *Journal of the History of Ideas* 61 (2000): 223–40.

Condliffe, Robin. "Merciful Release? A History of the British Voluntary Euthanasia Movement," B.Sc. diss., Wellcome Institute for the History of Medicine, 1995.

Conkin, Paul K. *When All the Gods Trembled: Darwinism, Scopes, and American Intellectuals.* Lanham, Md.: Rowman and Littlefield, 1998.

Cooney, John. *The American Pope: The Life and Times of Francis Cardinal Spellman.* New York: Times Books, 1984,

Critchlow, Donald T. *Intended Consequences: Birth Control, Abortion, and the Federal Government in Modern America.* New York: Oxford University Press, 1999.

———, ed. *The Politics of Abortion and Birth Control in Historical Perspective.* University Park: Pennsylvania State University Press, 1996.

Crocker, Lester G. "The Discussion of Suicide in the Eighteenth Century," *Journal of the History of Ideas* 13 (1952): 47–72.

Darwin, Charles. *The Origin of Species by Means of Natural Selection or the Preservation of Favoured Races in the Struggle for Life* (New York: Avenel Books, 1979), 458.

Degler, Carl N. *In Search of Human Nature: The Decline and Revival of Darwinism in American Social Thought.* New York: Oxford University Press, 1991.

Dewey, John. *Individualism, Old and New.* New York: Milton, Balch, 1930.

Dolan, Jay P. *The American Catholic Experience: A History from Colonial Times to the Present.* Garden City, N.Y.: Doubleday, 1985.

Dowbiggin, Ian R. *Keeping America Sane: Psychiatry and Eugenics in the United States and Canada, 1880–1940.* Ithaca, N.Y.: Cornell University Press, 1997.

———. " 'A Prey on Normal People': C. Killick Millard and the Euthanasia Movement in Great Britain, 1930–1955," *Journal of Contemporary History* 36 (2001): 59–85.

Downing, A. B., ed. *Euthanasia and the Right to Death: The Case for Voluntary Euthanasia.* London: Peter Owen, 1969.

Dugdale, R. L. *"The Jukes": A Study in Crime, Pauperism, and Heredity.* 4th ed. New York: Putnam, 1910.

Duster, Troy. *Backdoor to Eugenics.* New York: Routledge, 1990.

Elks, Martin A. "The 'Lethal Chamber': Further Evidence for the Euthanasia Option," *Mental Retardation* 31 (1993): 201–7.

Emanuel, Ezekiel J. "Euthanasia: Historical, Ethical, and Empiric Perspectives," *Archives of Internal Medicine* 154 (1994): 1890–1901.

————. "The History of Euthanasia Debates in the United States and Britain," *Annals of Internal Medicine* 121 (1994): 793–802.

Engel, Robert E. "Willystine Goodsell: Feminist and Reconstructionist Educator," *Vitae Scholasticae* 3 (1984): 355–78.

Engelhardt Jr., H. Tristam, and Edmund L. Erde. "Euthanasia in Texas: A Little Known Experiment," *Hospital Physician* 9 (1976): 30–31.

Filene, Peter G. *In the Arms of Others: A Cultural History of the Right-to-Die in America.* Chicago: Ivan Dee, 1998.

Fletcher, Joseph. *Morals and Medicine: The Moral Problems of: The Patient's Right to Know the Truth, Contraception, Artificial Insemination, Sterilization, Euthanasia.* 2d. ed. Princeton: Princeton University Press, 1979.

Foley, Kathleen, and Herbert Hendin, eds. *The Case Against Assisted Suicide: For the Right to End-of-Life Care.* Baltimore: Johns Hopkins University Press, 2002.

Fosdick, Harry Emerson. *Christianity and Progress.* New York and Chicago: Fleming H. Revell, 1922.

————. *The Living of These Days: An Autobiography.* New York: Harper and Brothers, 1956.

Friedlander, Henry. *The Origin of Nazi Genocide: From Euthanasia to the Final Solution.* Chapel Hill: University of North Carolina Press, 1995.

Friedman, George Alexander. "Suicide, Euthanasia, and the Law," *Medical Times* 85 (1957): 681–89.

Fye, W. Bruce "Active Euthanasia: An Historical Survey of its Conceptual Origins and Introduction into Medical Thought," *Bulletin of the History of Medicine* 52 (1979): 492–502.

Gallup, George H. *The Gallup Poll: Public Opinion, 1935–1971.* 3 vols. New York: Random House, 1972.

Gannon, Robert I. *The Cardinal Spellman Story.* Garden City, N.Y.: Doubleday, 1962.

Garrett, Valery. "The Last Civil Right? Euthanasia Policy and Politics in the United States, 1938–1991." Ph.D. diss., University of California at Santa Barbara, 1998.

Garrow, David J. *Liberty and Sexuality: The Right of Privacy and the Making of Roe v. Wade.* New York: Macmillan, 1994.

Glick, Henry R. *The Right to Die: Policy Innovation and Its Consequences.* New York: Columbia University Press, 1992.

Gordon, Linda. *Woman's Body, Woman's Right: A Social History of Birth Control in America.* Harmondsworth, Eng.: Penguin, 1977.

Gottfried, Paul Edward. *After Liberalism: Mass Democracy in the Managerial State.* Princeton: Princeton University Press, 1999.

Gourevitch, Danielle. "Suicide Among the Sick in Classical Antiquity," *Bulletin of the History of Medicine* 43 (1969): 501–18.

Graham, Otis L. *The Great Campaigns: Reform and War in America, 1900–1928.* Englewood Cliffs, N.J.: Prentice-Hall, 1971.

Green, Peter. *The Problem of Right Conduct: A Text-Book of Christian Ethics.* London and New York: Longmans, Green and Co., 1931.

Greene, John C. "Darwin as a Social Evolutionist," *Journal of the History of Biology* 10 (1977): 1–27.

Grisez, Germain, and Joseph M. Boyle Jr. *Life and Death with Liberty and Justice: A Contribution to the Euthanasia Debate.* Notre Dame: University of Notre Dame Press, 1979.

Gruman, Gerald J. "An Historical Introduction to Ideas about Voluntary Euthanasia: With a Bibliographic Survey and Guide for Interdisciplinary Studies," *Omega* 4 (1973): 87–138.

Haller, Mark H. *Eugenics: Hereditarian Attitudes in American Thought.* 2d ed. New Brunswick, N.J.: Rutgers University Press, 1984.

Harp, Gillis J. *Positivist Republic: Auguste Comte and the Reconstruction of American Liberalism, 1865–1920.* University Park: Pennsylvania State University Press, 1995.

Hawkins, Mike. *Social Darwinism in European and American Thought, 1860–1945.* Cambridge: Cambridge University Press, 1993.

Hays, Samuel P. *Conservation and the Gospel of Efficiency: The Progressive Conservation Movement.* Cambridge: Harvard University Press, 1959.

Heifetz, Louis J. "From Munchausen to Cassandra: A Critique of Hollander's 'Euthanasia and Mental Retardation,' " *Mental Retardation* 27 (1989): 67–69.

Helme, Tim. "The Voluntary Euthanasia (Legislation) Bill (1936) Revisited," *Journal of Medical Ethics* 17 (1991): 25–29.

Hofstadter, Richard. *The Age of Reform: From Bryan to F.D.R.* New York: Vintage, 1955.

———. *Social Darwinism in American Thought.* Rev. ed. Boston: Beacon Press, 1955.

Hollander, Russell. "Euthanasia and Mental Retardation: Suggesting the Unthinkable," *Mental Retardation* 27 (1989): 53–61.

Holmes, John Haynes. *The Revolutionary Function of the Modern Church.* New York: Putnam's, 1912.

Holmes, S. J. *Life and Morals.* New York: Macmillan, 1948.

Horan, Dennis J., and David Mall, eds. *Death, Dying, and Euthanasia.* Washington, D.C.: University Publications of America, 1977.

Hudson, Robert P. "The Many Faces of Euthanasia," *Medical Heritage* 2 (1986): 102–7.

Humphry, Derek, and Mary Clement. *Freedom to Die: People, Politics, and the Right-to-Die Movement.* New York: St. Martin's Griffin, 2000.

Humphry, Derek, and Ann Wickett. *The Right to Die: Understanding Euthanasia.* London: The Bodley Head, 1986.

Hutchison, William. *The Modernist Impulse in American Protestantism.* Cambridge: Harvard University Press. 1976.

Huxley, Julian. *Essays of a Humanist.* New York and Evanston: Harper and Row, 1964.

Irving, Allan. *Brock Chisholm: Doctor to the World.* Markham, Ontario: Fitzhenry and Whiteside, 1998.

Jalland, Pat. *Death in the Victorian Family.* New York: Oxford University Press, 1996.

Jones, James H. *Alfred C. Kinsey: A Public/Private Life*. New York: W. W. Norton, 1997.

Kallen, Horace M. "An Ethic of Freedom: A Philosopher's View," *New York University Law Review* 31 (1956): 1164–69.

Kamisar, Yale. "Some Non-Religious Views Against Proposed 'Mercy-Killing' Legislation," *Minnesota Law Review* 42 (1958): 969–1042.

Kaplan, Ronald P. "Euthanasia Legislation: A Survey and a Model Act," *American Journal of Law and Medicine* 2 (1976): 41–99.

Kater, Michael H. *Doctors Under Hitler*. Chapel Hill: University of North Carolina Press, 1989.

Kemp, Nicholas. "What Was the Nature of the Debate on Euthanasia in Great Britain Leading up to the Reading of the Voluntary Euthanasia (Legislation) Bill in December 1936?" Master's thesis, London School of Economics, 1995.

Kennedy, David M. *Birth Control in America: The Career of Margaret Sanger*. New Haven: Yale University Press, 1971.

Kevles, Daniel J. *In the Name of Eugenics: Genetics and the Uses of Human Heredity*. New York: Knopf, 1985.

Krutch, Joseph Wood. *The Modern Temper*. New York: Harcourt, Brace and Co., 1929.

Kübler-Ross, Elisabeth. *On Death and Dying*. New York: Macmillan, 1969.

Kuepper, Stephen Louis. "Euthanasia in America, 1890–1960: The Controversy, the Movement, and the Law." Ph.D. diss., Rutgers University, 1981.

Kühl, Stefan. *The Nazi Connection: Eugenics, American Racism, and German National Socialism*. New York: Oxford University Press, 1994.

Kushner, Howard I. "American Psychiatry and the Cause of Suicide, 1844–1917," *Bulletin of the History of Medicine* 60 (1986): 36–57.

———. *Self-Destruction in the Promised Land: A Psychocultural Biology of American Suicide*. New Brunswick, N.J.: Rutgers University Press, 1989.

Lader, Lawrence. *Politics, Power, and the Church: The Catholic Crisis and its Challenge to American Pluralism*. New York: Macmillan, 1987.

Landman, J. H. *Human Sterilization: A History of the Sexual Sterilization Movement*. New York: Macmillan, 1932.

Larson, Edward J. "Belated Progress: The Enactment of Eugenic Legislation in Georgia," *Journal of the History of Medicine and Allied Sciences* 46 (1991): 44–64.

———. *Sex, Race, and Science: Eugenics in the Deep South*. Baltimore: Johns Hopkins University Press, 1995.

———. *Summer for the Gods: The Scopes Trial and America's Continuing Debate Over Science and Religion*. New York: Basic Books, 1997.

Larson, Edward J., and Darrel W. Amundsen. *A Different Death: Euthanasia and the Christian Tradition*. Downers Grove, Ill.: InterVarsity Press, 1998.

Larue, Gerald A. *Euthanasia and Religion: A Survey of the Attitudes of World Religions to the Right-to-Die*. Los Angeles: The Hemlock Society, 1985.

Lowenberg, Bert James. "Darwinism Comes to America, 1859–1900," *Mississippi Valley Historical Review* 28 (1941): 339–68.

Ludmerer, Kenneth M. *Genetics and American Society: A Historical Appraisal.* Baltimore: Johns Hopkins University Press, 1972

Mannes, Marya. *Last Rights.* New York: William Morrow and Co., 1974.

Marker, Rita. *Deadly Compassion: The Death of Ann Humphry and the Case Against Euthanasia.* London: HarperCollins Publishers, 1993.

Marker, Rita L., et al., "Euthanasia: A Historical Overview," *Maryland Journal of Contemporary Legal Issues* 2 (1991): 257–98.

Marrus, Michael R. "The Nuremberg Doctors' Trial in Historical Context," *Bulletin of the History of Medicine* 73 (1999): 106–23.

McCann, Carole R. *Birth Control Politics in the United States, 1916–1945.* Ithaca, N.Y.: Cornell University Press, 1999.

McClay, Wilfred M. *The Masterless: Self and Society in Modern America.* Chapel Hill: University of North Carolina Press, 1994.

McGreevy, John T. "Thinking on One's Own: Catholicism in the American Intellectual Imagination, 1928–1960," *The Journal of American History* 84 (1997): 97–131.

McKim, W. Duncan. *Heredity and Human Progress.* New York: G. P. Putnam and Sons, 1900.

Mehler, Barry Alan. "A History of the American Eugenics Society, 1921–1940." Ph.D. diss., University of Illinois, Urbana-Champaign, 1988.

Miller, Robert Moats. *American Protestantism and Social Issues, 1919–1939.* Chapel Hill: University of North Carolina Press, 1958.

Minois, Georges. *History of Suicide: Voluntary Death in Western Culture.* Trans. Lydia G. Cochrane. Baltimore: Johns Hopkins University Press, 1999.

Moore, James R. *The Post-Darwinian Controversies: A Study of the Protestant Struggle to Come to Terms with Darwin in Great Britain and America, 1870–1900.* Cambridge: Cambridge University Press, 1979.

Moreno, Jonathan D., ed. *Arguing Euthanasia: The Controversy over Mercy-Killing, Assisted Suicide, and the "Right to Die."* New York: Simon and Schuster, 1995.

Morris, Charles R. *American Catholic: The Saints and Sinners Who Built America's Most Powerful Church.* New York: Times Books, 1997.

Neary, Peter, and Shaun Brown. "The Veterans Charter and Canadian Women Veterans of the Second World War," *British Journal of Canadian Studies* 9 (1994): 249–77.

The New York State Task Force on Life and the Law. *When Death Is Sought: Assisted Suicide and Euthanasia in the Medical Context.* New York, 1994.

Nuland, Sherwin B. *How We Die: Reflections on Life's Final Chapter.* New York: Knopf, 1994.

Numbers, Ronald L. *Darwinism Comes to America.* Cambridge: Harvard University Press, 1998.

Ostheimer, John M. "The Polls: Changing Attitudes Toward Euthanasia," *Public Opinion Quarterly* 44 (1980): 123–28.

Otlowski, Margaret. *Voluntary Euthanasia and the Common Law.* Oxford: Clarendon Press, 1997.

Pappas, Demetra M. "Recent Historical Perspectives Regarding Medical Euthanasia and Physician Assisted Suicide," *British Medical Bulletin* 52 (1996): 386–93.

Patterson, James T. *America in the Twentieth Century: A History.* Fort Worth, Tex.: Harcourt Brace, 1994.

———. *The Dread Disease: Cancer and Modern American Culture.* Cambridge: Harvard University Press, 1987.

Paul, Diane B. *Controlling Heredity: 1865 to the Present.* Atlantic Highlands, N.J.: Humanities Press, 1995.

Pernick, Martin S. *The Black Stork: Eugenics and the Death of "Defective" Babies in American Medicine and Motion Pictures Since 1915.* New York: Oxford University Press, 1996.

———. "Brain Death in a Cultural Context: The Reconstruction of Death, 1967–1981." In *The Definition of Death: Contemporary Controversies*, ed. Stuart Younger, Robert M. Arnold, and Renie Shapiro. Baltimore: Johns Hopkins University Press, 1999, 3–33.

———. "Eugenic Euthanasia in Early Twentieth-Century America and Medically Assisted Suicide Today: Differences and Similarities." In *Law at the End of Life: The Supreme Court and Assisted Suicide*, ed. Carl E. Schneider, 221–38. Ann Arbor: University of Michigan Press, 2000.

———. "Eugenics and Public Health in American History," *American Journal of Public Health* 87, no. 11 (1997): 1767–72.

Pickens, Donald K. *Eugenics and the Progressives.* Nashville: Vanderbilt University Press, 1969.

Porter, Roy. *The Greatest Benefit to Mankind: A Medical History of Humanity.* New York: W. W. Norton and Co., 1998.

Potter, Charles Francis. *Creative Personality: The Next Step in Evolution.* New York: Funk and Wagnalls, 1950.

———. *The Preacher and I: An Autobiography.* New York: Crown Publishers, 1951.

Proctor, Robert N. *The Nazi War on Cancer.* Princeton: Princeton University Press, 1999.

———. *Racial Hygiene: Medicine Under the Nazis.* Cambridge: Harvard University Press, 1988.

Quill, Timothy E. *Caring for Patients at the End of Life: Facing an Uncertain Future Together.* New York: Oxford University Press, 2001.

Rafter, Nicole Hahn. *Creating Born Criminals.* Urbana: University of Illinois Press, 1997.

Ramsey, Paul. *Ethics at the Edges of Life: Medical and Legal Intersections.* New Haven: Yale University Press, 1978.

Rattray, Robert Fleming. *From Primitive to Modern Religion.* London: Lindsey Press, 1937.

———. "The Right to Painless Death," *Quarterly Review* 274 (1940): 39–49.

Reed, James. *From Private Vice to Public Virtue: The Birth Control Movement and American Society Since 1830.* New York: Basic Books, 1978.

Reilly, Philip R. *The Surgical Solution: A History of Involuntary Sterilization in the United States.* Baltimore: Johns Hopkins University Press, 1991.

Robinson, David. *The Unitarians and the Universalists.* Westport, Conn.: Greenwood Press, 1985.

Robinson, Victor, ed. "A Symposium on Euthanasia," *Medical Review of Reviews* 19 (1913): 134–55.

Robinson, William J. "Euthanasia," *Medico-Pharmaceutical Critic and Guide* 16 (1913): 85–90.

Rosenberg, Charles E. *The Care of Strangers: The Rise of America's Hospital System.* New York: Basic Books, 1987.

Ross, Dorothy. *The Origins of American Social Science.* Cambridge: Cambridge University Press, 1991.

Ross, Dorothy, ed. *Modernist Impulses in the Human Sciences, 1870–1930.* Baltimore: Johns Hopkins University Press, 1994.

Rothman, David J. *Conscience and Convenience: The Asylum and Its Alternatives in Progressive America.* Boston: Little, Brown, 1980.

———. *Strangers at the Bedside: A History of How Law and Bioethics Transformed Medical Decision-Making.* New York: Basic Books, 1992.

Ruse, Michael. *The Darwinian Revolution: Science Red in Tooth and Claw.* Chicago: University of Chicago Press, 1979.

Russell, Olive Ruth. *Freedom to Die: Moral and Legal Aspects of Euthanasia.* Rev. ed. New York: Human Sciences Press, 1977.

Russett, Cynthia Eagle. *Darwin in America: The Intellectual Response, 1865–1912.* San Francisco: W. H. Freeman, 1976.

Sandburg, Carl. *The People, Yes.* New York: Harcourt Brace and World, 1936.

Sanger, Margaret, ed. *The Sixth International Neo-Malthusian and Birth Control Conference.* Vol 2. New York: The American Birth Control League, 1926.

Shapiro, Thomas M. *Population Control Politics: Women, Sterilization, and Reproductive Choice.* Philadelphia: Temple University Press, 1985.

Sharpless, John. "World Population Growth, Family Planning, and American Foreign Policy." In *The Politics of Abortion and Birth Control in Historical Perspective,* ed. Donald T. Critchlow, 72–102. University Park: Pennsylvania State University Press, 1996.

Shorter, Edward. *Bedside Manners: The Troubled History of Doctors and Patients.* New York: Simon and Schuster, 1985.

Slome, Lee R., et al. "Physician-Assisted Suicide and Patients with Human Immunodeficiency Virus Disease," *New England Journal of Medicine* 336 (1997): 417–21.

Smith, Wesley J. *Forced Exit: The Slippery Slope from Assisted Suicide to Legalized Murder.* New York: Times Books, 1997.

Soloway, Richard A. *Birth Control and the Population Question in England, 1877–1930.* Chapel Hill: University of North Carolina Press, 1982.

———. *Demography and Degeneration: Eugenics and the Declining Birthrate in Twentieth-Century Britain.* 2d ed. Chapel Hill: University of North Carolina Press, 1995.

Stannard, David E., ed. *Death in America.* Philadelphia: University of Pennsylvania Press, 1975.

Starr, Paul. *The Social Transformation of American Medicine.* New York: Basic Books, 1982.

Steinfels, Peter, and Robert M. Veatch, eds. *Death Inside Out: The Hastings Center Report.* New York: Harper and Row, 1975.

Stepan, Nancy Leys. *"The Hour of Eugenics": Race, Gender, and Nation in Latin America.* Ithaca, N.Y.: Cornell University Press, 1991.

Swallow, Susan Ruth. "Olive Ruth Russell: A Twentieth-Century Canadian Progressive." Master's thesis, University of Western Ontario, 1996.

Thomas, Lewis. "Dying as Failure," *Annals of the American Academy of Political and Social Science* 447 (1980): 1–4.

Tomkins, Jerry R., ed. *D-Days at Dayton: Reflections on the Scopes Trail.* Baton Rouge: Louisiana State University Press, 1965.

Van Der Sluis, I. "The Movement for Euthanasia, 1875–1975," *Janus* 66 (1979): 131–72.

Vanessendelft, William Ray. "A History of the Association for Voluntary Sterilization, 1935–1964." Ph.D. diss., University of Minnesota, 1978.

Veatch, Robert M. "Medical Ethics in the Soviet Union," *Hastings Center Report* 19 (1989): 11–14.

Vecoli, Rudolph J. "Sterilization: A Progressive Measure?" *Wisconsin Magazine of History* 43 (1960): 190–202.

Vogel, Morris J., and Charles E. Rosenberg, eds. *The Therapeutic Revolution: Essays in the Social History of American Medicine.* Philadelphia: University of Pennsylvania Press, 1979.

Vovelle, Michel. "Rediscovery of Death Since 1960," *Annals of the American Academy of Political and Social Science* 447 (1980): 89–99.

Wakefield, Eva Ingersoll, ed. *The Letters of Robert G. Ingersoll.* New York: Philosophical Library, 1951.

Weikart, Richard. "Darwinism and Death: Devaluing Human Life in Germany, 1859–1918." Paper presented at the West Coast History of Science Society, University of California, Berkeley, May 2000.

Weindling, Paul. *Health, Race and German Politics Between National Unification and Nazism, 1870–1945.* Cambridge: Cambridge University Press, 1989.

Wertenbaker, Lael. *Death of a Man.* Boston: Beacon Press, 1957.

Wiebe, Robert H. *The Search for Order, 1877–1920.* New York: Hill and Wang, 1967.

Wiggam, Albert E. *The New Decalogue of Science.* Indianapolis: Bobbs-Merrill, 1923.

Williams, Glanville. "Euthanasia and Abortion," *University of Colorado Law Review* 38 (1966): 178–201.

———. *The Sanctity of Life and the Criminal Law.* New York: Knopf, 1968.

Williams, Samuel D. "Euthanasia," *Popular Science Monthly* 3 (1873): 90–96.

Woodman, Sue. *Last Rights: The Struggle Over the Right to Die.* New York: Plenum, 1998.

Younger, Stuart J., Robert M. Arnold, and Renie Schapiro, eds. *The Definition of Death: Contemporary Controversies.* Baltimore: Johns Hopkins University Press, 1999.

Zenderland, Leila. "Biblical Biology: American Protestant Social Reformers and the Early Eugenics Movement" *Science in Context* 11 (1998).

Zucker, Marjorie B., ed. *The Right to Die Debate: A Documentary History.* Westport, Conn.: Greenwood Press, 1999.

Index

and Hugh Moore's bequest, 144–45; merger with Concern for Dying, 160–62; relations with Concern for Dying in the 1980s, 154–62; split with Concern for Dying, 140–45

Spellman, Francis Cardinal, 83, 91, 92, 99–100

Spencer, Herbert, 9, 14, 20, 21

Standish, Hilda Crosby, 80

Stout, Rex, 52

Straton, John Roach, 39–40

Suicide, incidence of, 34, 152–53, 188 n. 90

Sumner, William Graham, 14

Supreme Court (U.S.), xviii, 163, 164–65, 170, 172

Taussig, Helen, 147, 159, 213 n. 115

Taylor, Pauline, 107–8, 142

Terminal sedation, 175

Texas. *See* Euthanasia: in Texas

Thalidomide disaster, 97, 111, 209 n. 56

Thanatology, 117

Tocqueville, Alexis de, 2, 111

Tompkins, Jean Burnett, 72, 198 n. 23

Torcaso, Roy, 214 n. 120

Toynbee, Arnold, 112

Transcendentalism, 42

Tredgold, A. F., 190 n. 12

The Truth Seeker, 90, 91

Union Theological Seminary, 85, 86, 88, 131, 202 n. 69

Unitarian Universalist Association, 129, 168, 172

Unitarianism, 41–42, 43–44, 52, 73, 79, 85, 108, 120, 124, 129–30, 138. *See also* Euthanasia: and Unitarianism

United Nations Commission on the Status of Women, 79

University of Nebraska School of Pharmacy, 49

Van Dusen, Henry P., 86, 131, 216 n. 140

Van Vleck, Louise, 157, 160. *See also* Moore, Louise Wilde

Visher, Stephen S., 54

Vogt, William, 130

Voltaire, 3

Voluntary Euthanasia Legislation Society, 51–52, 57, 59, 63, 71, 72, 79, 81, 95, 104, 105; change of name to EXIT, 149; change of name to the Voluntary Euthanasia Society, 149

Voluntary Euthanasia Society, 149

Voluntary Euthanasia Society of Connecticut, 80

Wakefield, Eva Ingersoll, 41

Wald, Lillian, 26

Wanzer, Sidney, 159

Washington Citizens for Death With Dignity, 168

Washington Physicians Against 119, 170

Washington State, vote on euthanasia in, 167–70

Washington State Medical Association, 170

Washington v. Glucksberg, 173

Wasserman, Richard, 157, 160, 161, 165

"Wedge" theory, 28, 93, 105–6, 156

Wells, H. G., 52, 54

Wertenbaker, Lael, 110, 208 n. 45

Wesley, John, 3–4

Whelpton, P. K., 130

When Death Is Sought, 174

Whitney, Leon F., 54

Wickett, Ann, 149, 151